About the NCCN Guidelines for Patients®

National Comprehensive Cancer Network®

AF824555

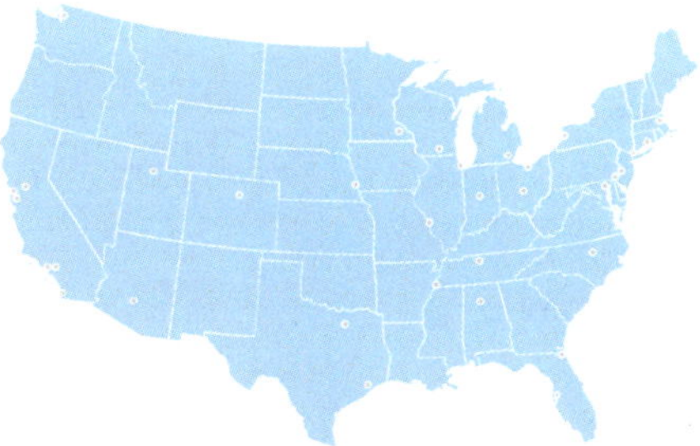

Did you know that top cancer centers across the United States work together to improve cancer care? This alliance of leading cancer centers is called the National Comprehensive Cancer Network® (NCCN®).

Cancer care is always changing. NCCN develops evidence-based cancer care recommendations used by health care providers worldwide. These frequently updated recommendations are the NCCN Clinical Practice Guidelines in Oncology (NCCN Guidelines®). The NCCN Guidelines for Patients plainly explain these expert recommendations for people with cancer and caregivers.

These NCCN Guidelines for Patients are based on the NCCN Clinical Practice Guidelines in Oncology (NCCN Guidelines®) for Kidney Cancer, Version 2.2025 – September 6, 2024.

View the NCCN Guidelines for Patients free online
NCCN.org/patientguidelines

Find an NCCN Cancer Center near you
NCCN.org/cancercenters

Connect with us

Supporters

NCCN Guidelines for Patients are supported by funding from the NCCN Foundation®

NCCN Foundation gratefully acknowledges the following corporate supporters for helping to make available these NCCN Guidelines for Patients: Bristol Myers Squibb; Eisai, Inc.; and Exelixis, Inc.

NCCN independently adapts, updates, and hosts the NCCN Guidelines for Patients. Our corporate supporters do not participate in the development of the NCCN Guidelines for Patients and are not responsible for the content and recommendations contained therein.

To make a gift or learn more, visit online or email

NCCNFoundation.org/donate

PatientGuidelines@NCCN.org

Contents

NCCN Foundation seeks to support the millions of patients and their families affected by a cancer diagnosis by funding and distributing NCCN Guidelines for Patients. NCCN Foundation is also committed to advancing cancer treatment by funding the nation's promising doctors at the center of innovation in cancer research. For more details and the full library of patient and caregiver resources, visit NCCN.org/patients.

National Comprehensive Cancer Network (NCCN) and NCCN Foundation
3025 Chemical Road, Suite 100, Plymouth Meeting, PA 19462 USA

1
About kidney cancer

The kidneys are a pair of organs found behind the other organs in your abdomen. The kidneys make hormones and filter blood to remove waste and extra water from the body. This chapter will discuss the kidneys and provide an overview of kidney cancer.

The kidneys

The kidneys are a pair of organs found behind the other organs in your abdomen. Each kidney is about the size of an adult's fist. The kidney is covered by a thin layer of tissue, like the skin of an apple. This layer of tissue is called the renal capsule. Renal refers to the kidney.

The kidneys are part of the urinary system. The urinary system is a group of organs that remove waste from the body in the form of urine (or pee). This system includes the kidneys, ureters, bladder, and urethra. The kidneys make hormones that help control blood pressure. They also make hormones that tell the body to make more red blood cells. By filtering the blood, the kidneys also control and balance the levels of fluids and chemicals in your body.

The kidneys and urinary system

The kidneys are the main organs of the urinary system. The ureters, bladder, and urethra hold and transport urine before it is released from the body.

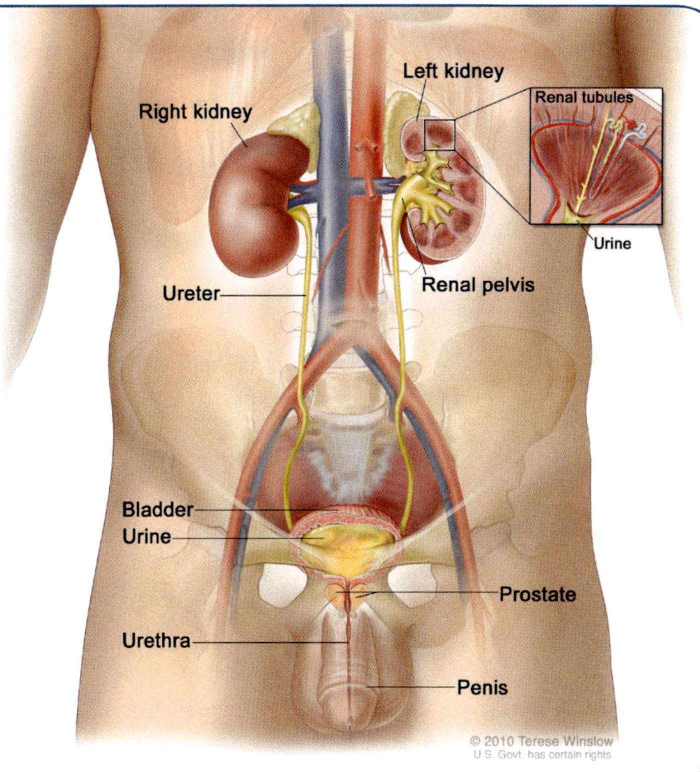

An adrenal gland sits on top of each kidney. The kidney and adrenal gland are surrounded by a layer of fat. Covering the fat is an outer layer of fibrous tissue called Gerota's fascia. When kidney cancer grows into and beyond Gerota's fascia, it is a sign of advanced kidney cancer.

How the kidneys work

The kidneys perform many jobs to keep your body healthy. The main job of the kidneys is to filter blood to remove waste and extra water from the body. By filtering the blood, the kidneys also control and balance the levels of fluids and chemicals in your body.

The renal artery carries blood with waste into the kidney. Blood then flows through tiny filtering tubes in the kidney called renal tubules. Blood is cleaned as it flows through the renal tubules. The renal tubules remove waste and other substances from the blood. These substances are made into urine.

The clean, filtered blood flows out of the kidney through the renal vein. The renal vein merges with a larger vein called the vena cava. The vena cava takes clean blood back up to the heart.

Urine flows out of the renal tubules and collects in a hollow space in the middle of the kidney called the renal pelvis. Urine leaves the renal pelvis through a long tube called the

The kidneys filter blood to remove waste

Blood enters the kidney through the renal artery. Renal tubules remove excess water and other waste from the blood to make urine. Urine drips out of the renal tubules into the renal pelvis, then leaves the kidney through the ureter. Clean, filtered blood leaves the kidney through the renal vein.

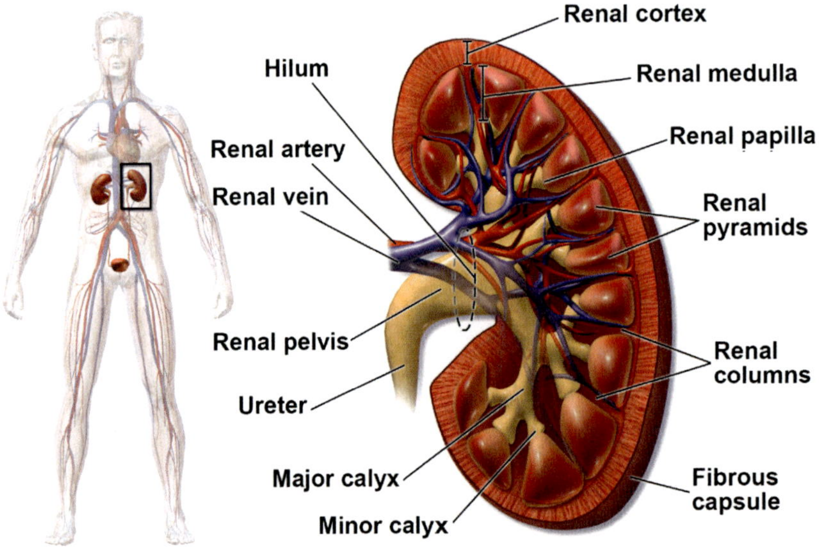

ureter. The ureter carries urine to the bladder. The bladder holds urine until it is released from the body when you urinate (or pee). A shorter tube, called the urethra, takes urine from the bladder to outside the body.

Most people have two kidneys. However, each kidney works on its own and does not need the other to function. This means that the body can often work well with less than one complete kidney. Many people live full, healthy lives with only one kidney.

Kidney cancer

Kidney cancer starts in the tissues of the kidneys. Almost all kidney cancers are carcinomas. Carcinomas are cancers that start in cells that line the inner or outer surfaces of the body. In the kidneys, carcinomas most often start in the cells that line the renal tubules. This is called renal cell carcinoma (RCC). About 9 out of 10 kidney cancers are RCCs. RCC may appear as multiple tumors in one kidney or involve both kidneys. Because it is the most common type, RCC is often simply referred to as kidney cancer. RCC is the focus of this book.

There are other, less common cancers that can arise in the kidney. While they can sometimes be confused with RCC, it is important to note that they are treated differently.

- **Urothelial carcinoma** starts in the cells that line the renal pelvis and ureter that drain the kidney. While these tumors can be found up the ureter near the kidneys, they are not kidney tumors. These tumors share many features with bladder cancer. These tumors used to be called transitional call cancer. For more information, see *NCCN Guidelines for Patients: Bladder Cancer*, available at NCCN.org/patientguidelines and on the NCCN Patient Guides for Cancer app.
- **Wilms tumor (nephroblastoma)** usually occurs in young children. In Wilms tumor (WT), cancer cells are found in the kidney.
- **Renal sarcoma** starts in the blood vessels or connective tissue of the kidney. For more information, see *NCCN Guidelines for Patients: Soft Tissue Sarcoma*, available at NCCN.org/patientguidelines and on the NCCN Patient Guides for Cancer app.

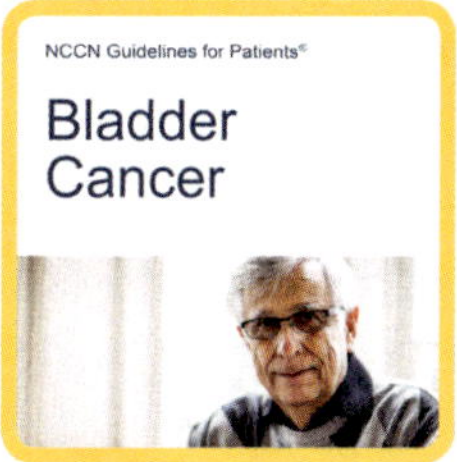

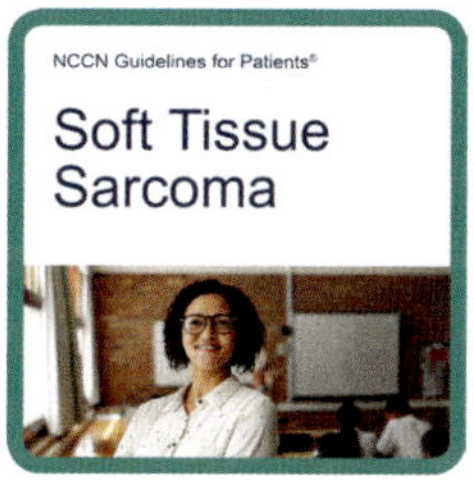

RCC subtypes

Renal cell carcinoma (RCC) is the most common type of kidney cancer. RCC can be broken down into subtypes by looking at the cancer cells under a microscope. This is called histology. Tumor histology and other factors are an important part of choosing a treatment plan. Ask your care team about your cancer subtype.

Clear cell RCC

Clear cell RCC (ccRCC) is the most common subtype. It occurs in about 7 out of 10 people with RCC. Under a microscope, clear cells look very pale or clear.

Non-clear cell RCC

Non-clear cell RCC is also called nccRCC There are several subtypes.

- **Papillary RCC** is the most common subtype of nccRCC (about 1 out of 10 people with RCC). Most papillary tumors look like long, thin finger-like growths under a microscope. It is also called PRCC.
- **Chromophobe RCC** cells are pale, but larger than clear cells, and look different.

Rare types of nccRCC

Other rare types of nccRCC include the following:

- **Collecting duct RCC (cdRCC)** forms in the cells of the collecting ducts or tubules.
- **Renal medullary carcinoma (RMC)** can be found in young people of African descent who carry the sickle cell trait, sickle cell disease, or other diseases that can cause sickling of the red blood cells.
- **Translocation RCC** can be found at all ages but tends to be diagnosed in children or younger adults. These tumors have unique fusions of genes that promote the cancer.
- **Unclassified RCC** describes cancer cells that don't look like any of the subtypes or more than one subtype is present.

Some other RCC types that have been defined recently include:

- Clear cell papillary renal cell tumor
- Fumarate hydratase-deficient RCC
- ELOC (formerly TCEB1)-mutated RCC

Renal cell carcinoma

Most kidney cancers arise in cells that line the small tubes in the kidney called renal tubules.

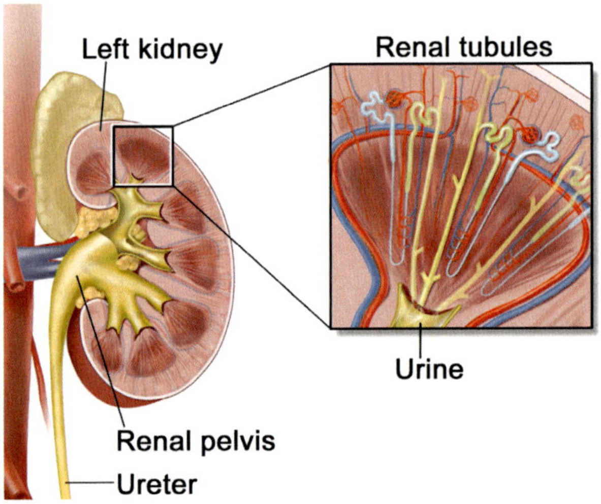

Sarcomatoid features

Almost any type of renal cell carcinoma can become sarcomatoid (sRCC) or have sarcomatoid features. This means that the cells of the cancer look like the cells of a sarcoma (cancer of the connective tissues, such as muscles, nerves, fat, blood vessels, and fibrous tissue). Sarcomatoid renal cancers occur in less than 10% of RCC tumors but when present tend to grow more quickly than other types of kidney cancer and are more likely to spread to other parts of the body. This makes them more difficult to treat.

How kidney cancer spreads

Tumors can grow in any part of the kidney and can grow into the renal vein and vena cava. Kidney cancer can also spread to other parts of the body in a process called metastasis. In metastasis, cancer cells travel through your blood or lymph to form new tumors outside of the kidney. The new tumors are called metastatic tumors or metastases.

- **Local spread** – In locally advanced disease, cancer has spread to a nearby area close to the primary tumor. Kidney cancer can invade nearby tissues like surrounding fat, blood vessels, lymph nodes, adrenal glands, and Gerota's fascia.
- **Distant metastasis** – In metastatic disease, cancer has spread to distant parts of the body far from the primary site. Kidney cancer tends to spread to distant sites such as the lungs, lymph nodes, and bones, and less frequently to the liver and brain. Multiple tumors in one or both kidneys are not considered metastasis and are treated as separate primary tumors.

Treatment will be based on the size, known or suspected subtype, and location of the tumor(s).

Key points

- The kidneys filter blood to remove extra water and other waste the body doesn't need.
- Blood flows into the kidney through the renal artery and out through the renal vein.
- Renal tubules are tiny tubes in the kidneys that remove waste from blood and make urine.
- Renal cell carcinoma (RCC) starts in cells that line the renal tubules. RCC is the most common type of kidney cancer and is the focus of the book. Clear cell RCC and non-clear cell RCC are subtypes.
- Almost any type of RCC can become sarcomatoid (sRCC) or have sarcomatoid features.
- Tumors can grow in any part of the kidney and can grow into the renal vein and vena cava.
- Treatment for RCC is based on histology, tumor(s) size and location, and if cancer has metastasized to other areas in the body.

2

Diagnosing kidney cancer

Most kidney cancers are found by chance during imaging tests for other health problems. Further testing is used to confirm (diagnose) kidney cancer. This chapter presents an overview of possible tests you might receive and what to expect.

Test results

Results from imaging studies and possible biopsy will be used to determine your treatment plan. Treatment will be based on these findings. It is important you understand what these tests mean. Ask questions about your test results.

Keep these things in mind:

- It's beneficial to have a support system in place during diagnosis and treatment. Enlist the help of friends, family members, or peers who can provide transportation, meals, and emotional support. These can be different people for different tasks or change over time.
- Consider bringing someone with you to doctor visits if possible or have someone on the phone or join you for telehealth visits.
- Don't hesitate to ask questions and take notes during appointments. Write down questions and ask a friend or family member to take notes. Caregivers should ask questions, too.
- Organize your medical documents, including insurance forms, medical records, and test results. Keep a list of contact information for your care team and update your primary care physician (PCP) regarding any changes. Include details about the specific type of cancer, treatment, and dates in your contact list.
- Ask your care team how best to communicate with them, especially in an emergency.

For possible tests and procedures, **see Guide 1.**

Guide 1 Possible tests
Medical history and physical exam
Complete blood count, differential, comprehensive metabolic panel, lactate dehydrogenase
Urinalysis
CT or MRI scan of abdomen with or without pelvis.
Chest CT (preferred) or chest x-ray
As needed: bone scan, brain MRI, chest CT, core needle biopsy, or other tests
If multiple kidney masses, 46 years of age or under, or family history, possible genetic risk testing

General health tests

Some general health tests are described next.

Medical history

A medical history is a record of all health issues and treatments you have had in your life. Be prepared to list any illness or injury and when it happened. Bring a list of old and new medicines and any over-the-counter (OTC) medicines, herbals, or supplements you take. Some supplements interact with and affect medicines that your care team may prescribe. Tell your care team about any symptoms you have. A medical history, sometimes called a health history, will help determine which treatment is best for you.

Family history

Some cancers and other diseases can run in families. Your care team will ask about the health history of family members who are blood relatives. This information is called a family history. Ask family members on both sides of your family about their health issues like heart disease, cancer, and diabetes, and at what age they were diagnosed. It's important to know the specific type of cancer or where the cancer started, if it is in multiple locations, and if they had genetic testing.

Physical exam

During a physical exam, your health care provider may:

- Check your temperature, blood pressure, pulse, and breathing rate
- Check your height and weight
- Listen to your lungs and heart
- Look in your eyes, ears, nose, and throat
- Feel and apply pressure to parts of your body to see if organs are of normal size, are soft or hard, or cause pain when touched.
- Feel for enlarged lymph nodes in your neck, underarm, and groin.

Blood tests

Blood tests check for signs of disease and how well organs are working. They require a sample of your blood, which is removed through a needle placed into a vein in your arm. Some blood tests are described next.

Complete blood count and differential

A complete blood count (CBC) measures the levels of red blood cells (RBCs), white blood cells (WBCs), and platelets (PLTs) in your blood. Red blood cells carry oxygen throughout your body, white blood cells fight infection, and platelets control bleeding. A differential counts the number of each type of white blood cell. It also checks if the counts are in balance with each other.

Comprehensive metabolic panel

A comprehensive metabolic panel (CMP) measures substances in your blood. It is usually done on the plasma part of your blood. A CMP provides important information about how well your kidneys and liver are working, among other things. A CMP might include a serum creatinine test, liver function tests (LFTs), and a urinalysis. These tests might also be called blood chemistry tests.

Alkaline phosphatase

Alkaline phosphatase (ALP) is an enzyme found in the blood. High levels of ALP can be a sign cancer has spread to the bone or liver. A bone scan might be performed if you have high levels of ALP.

Calcium

Calcium is the most common mineral in the body. It is needed for healthy teeth, bones, and other body tissues. You might have higher calcium levels if your kidneys aren't working normally. Bone damage from cancer can cause your bones to release calcium into the bloodstream.

Creatinine

Creatinine is a waste produced in the muscles. Every person generates a fixed amount of creatinine every day based on how much muscle they have. It is filtered out of the blood by the kidneys. The level of creatinine in the blood tells how well the kidneys are working. Higher levels of creatinine mean the kidneys aren't working as well as they were when someone had lower levels of creatinine.

Lactate dehydrogenase

Lactate dehydrogenase (LDH) or lactic acid dehydrogenase is an enzyme found in most cells. Dying cells release LDH into the blood. Fast-growing cells, such as tumor cells, also release LDH.

Liver function tests

Liver function tests (LFTs) look at the health of your liver by measuring chemicals that are made or processed by the liver. Levels that are too high or low signal that the liver is not working well or that cancer has spread to the liver.

Urine tests

Urine tests look for signs of disease and assess your general health. Abnormal results may signal there's a problem with your kidneys or other organs. Abnormal results may be caused by kidney cancer or other health conditions. For a urine test, you will be asked to fill a small container with urine. The urine sample will be sent to a lab for testing.

Urinalysis

A urinalysis detects and/or measures several substances in the urine using a microscope and chemical tests. Blood in urine (hematuria) may be caused by kidney cancer or other health problems. Those with kidney cancer may have a normal urinalysis or have evidence of blood in the urine.

Urine cytology

In urine cytology, urine is looked at under a microscope to check for cancer cells. This test may be used if your care team suspects urothelial cancer in the urinary tract or bladder.

Imaging tests

Imaging tests take pictures of the inside of your body. Imaging tests show the primary tumor, or where the cancer started, and look for cancer in other parts of the body. A radiologist, an expert in interpreting imaging tests, will write a report and send this report to your health care provider (HCP). While these reports might be available to you through your patient portal or patient access system, please wait to discuss these results with your care team.

You will have some, but not all of the following tests. If you have questions about why a test is or isn't recommended, ask your HCP.

Contrast material

Contrast material is used to improve the pictures of the inside of the body. Contrast materials are substances that help enhance and improve the images of several organs and structures in the body. It is used to make the pictures clearer. The contrast is not permanent and will leave your body in your urine immediately after the test. The types of contrast vary and are different for CT and MRI.

Tell your care team if you have had allergic reactions to contrast in the past. This is important. You might be given medicines to avoid the effects of those allergies. Contrast might not be used if you have a serious allergy or if your kidneys aren't working well.

CT scan

A CT or CAT (computed tomography) scan uses x-rays and computer technology to take pictures of the inside of the body. It takes many x-rays of the same body part from different angles. All the images are combined to make one detailed picture. A CT scan of your chest, abdomen, and/or pelvis may be one of the tests to look for cancer. In most cases, contrast will be used.

MRI scan

An MRI (magnetic resonance imaging) scan uses radio waves and powerful magnets to take pictures of the inside of the body. It does not use x-rays. Because of the very strong magnets used in the MRI machine, tell the technologist if you have any metal in your body. During the test, you will likely be asked to hold your breath for 10 to 20 seconds as the technician collects the images. Contrast is often used.

A closed MRI has a capsule-like design where the magnet surrounds you. An open MRI has a magnetic top and bottom, which allows for an opening on each end. Closed MRIs are more common than open MRIs, so if you have claustrophobia (a dread or fear of enclosed spaces), be sure to talk to your care team about it.

MRI is most often used to evaluate the abdomen and pelvis, but may also be used to look at possible tumor spread (metastasis) in the brain.

Bone scan

Kidney cancer can spread to bones. A bone scan uses a radiotracer, a substance that releases small amounts of radiation. Before the pictures are taken, the tracer will be injected into your vein. It can take a few hours for the tracer to enter your bones. However, the test is quick and painless.

A special camera will take pictures of the tracer in your bones as it moves over your body. Areas of bone damage take up more radiotracer than healthy bone and show up as bright spots on the pictures. Bone damage can be caused by cancer, cancer treatment, previous injuries, or other health issues. This test may be used if you have bone pain, are at high risk for bone metastases, or if there are changes in certain test results. Bone scans might be used to monitor treatment.

Ultrasound

An ultrasound (US) uses high-energy sound waves to form pictures of the inside of the body. This is similar to the sonogram used for pregnancy. A wand-like probe (transducer) will be held and moved on your skin using gel. Ultrasound is painless and does not use x-rays, so it can be repeated as needed. An ultrasound can show if there is a mass in your kidney and if the mass is solid or fluid-filled. It can also help evaluate if the mass has blood flow. Kidney cancer tumors are more likely to be solid and have blood flow.

X-ray

An x-ray is a type of radiation. In small doses, it is used to make pictures of the inside of the body. A chest x-ray is used to see if cancer has spread to the lungs. It might be referred to as a radiograph.

The kidney and adrenal gland

An adrenal gland sits on top of each kidney. The kidney and adrenal gland are surrounded by a layer of fatty tissue. Surrounding the fat is a layer of fibrous tissue called Gerota's fascia.

Derivative work of Kidney and Adrenal Gland by Alan Hoofring from NCI Visuals Online. Available at: https://visualsonline.cancer.gov/details.cfm?imageid=4355

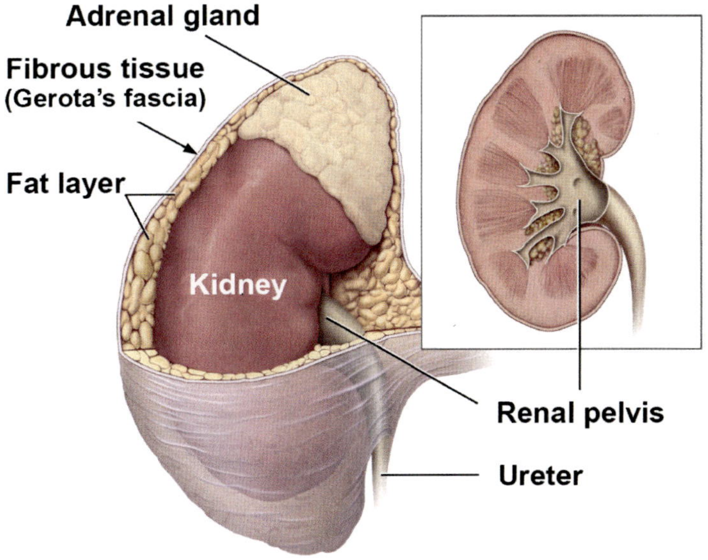

National Cancer Institute

Biopsy

A biopsy removes a sample of tissue or fluid. Samples removed during a biopsy or surgery will be sent to a pathologist, an expert in examining cells under a microscope to confirm the presence of cancer. The pathologist will determine the cancer subtype called tumor histology.

For most cancers, a biopsy must be done to confirm cancer before starting cancer treatment. However, for many with a high suspicion of kidney cancer that appears to be contained to the kidney, the primary treatment is surgery to remove the tumor. After the tumor is removed, it is tested (biopsied).

Other types of biopsies may include:

- **Fine-needle aspiration (FNA)** or fine needle biopsy (FNB) uses a thin needle to remove a sample of tissue or fluid. An ultrasound may guide the FNA biopsy.
- **Core needle biopsy (CNB)** removes tissue samples with a hollow needle about the same size as a needle used for an IV (intravenous) line.

Biopsy of metastases

Metastasis is the spread of cancer to an area of the body such as lung, bone, or brain. A biopsy of the metastasis may be needed to confirm the presence of cancer. If there is more than one metastasis, each site may be biopsied. The type of biopsy used depends on the location of the suspected metastases and other factors.

Biopsy results

Histology is the study of the anatomy (structure) of cells, tissues, and organs under a microscope. It is used to make treatment decisions. Your pathology report will contain information about histology

Biomarker testing

A sample from a biopsy of your tumor may be tested to look for specific DNA (deoxyribonucleic acid) mutations/alterations, protein levels, or other molecular features. It is sometimes called molecular testing or tumor profiling, tumor sequencing, gene expression profiling, or genomic testing. These tests are more commonly done in those with advanced disease to choose the best treatment for you.

Biomarker testing includes tests of genes or their products (proteins). Proteins are written like this: SDHB (which stands for Succinate Dehydrogenase Complex Iron Sulfur Subunit B). Genes are written with italics like this: *SDHB.*

Tumor mutation testing

Tumor mutation testing, tumor genomic aberration testing, or somatic testing uses a sample of your tumor or blood to see if the cancer cells have any specific DNA mutations. This is a different type of DNA testing than the genetic risk testing for mutations you may have inherited from your biological parents (called germline testing). In tumor mutation testing, only the tumor is tested. Some mutations can be targeted with specific therapies. These tests are more commonly done in those with advanced disease.

Genetic risk testing

You might be thinking why did I get cancer? Most of the time, the answer is one cell made a mistake when dividing and then a cancer formed. Some, however, have a predisposition or have something in their DNA (genetic material) that makes them more likely to develop cancer. Understanding whether you have a cancer predisposition condition can sometimes affect your cancer treatment, but more often, it can affect screening for other cancers. Therefore, identifying a cancer predisposition condition is important.

Genetic testing is done using blood or saliva (spitting into a cup or a cheek swab). The goal is to look for gene mutations inherited from your biological parents called germline mutations. Some mutations can put you at risk for more than one type of cancer. You can pass these genes on to your children. Also, family members might carry these mutations. Tell your care team if there is a family history of cancer.

Hereditary cancer predisposition syndromes

Certain genetic (inherited) syndromes may put someone at risk for developing kidney cancer. A syndrome is a group of signs or symptoms that occur together and suggest the presence of or risk for a disease. A hereditary syndrome is found in blood (biological) relatives.

A genetic risk assessment will identify if you carry a cancer risk and if you may benefit from genetic testing, additional screening, or preventive interventions. Depending on the genetic risk assessment, you might undergo genetic testing and genetic counseling to see if you have a hereditary syndrome that puts you at risk for developing kidney cancer, along with possibly other cancers or medical issues.

- **Hereditary renal cell carcinoma (HRCC)** is kidney cancer caused by a hereditary syndrome. More information on HRCC can be found in *Chapter 7: Hereditary RCC.*

It is important that those who have hereditary causes of RCC see their doctors often, especially if they have already been diagnosed with RCC. Those with confirmed hereditary causes of RCC will be monitored differently than those with sporadic RCC. You will have regular testing to check for a new kidney tumor and may also need follow up with other specialists depending on the type of hereditary RCC.

Performance status

Performance status (PS) is a person's general level of fitness and ability to perform daily tasks. Your state of general health will be rated using a PS scale called Eastern Cooperative Oncology Group (ECOG) or the Karnofsky Performance Score (KPS). PS is one factor taken into consideration when choosing a treatment plan. Your preferences about treatment are always important.

Key points

- Results from blood tests, imaging studies, and possible biopsy will determine your treatment plan. Often, information is collected over time, even as treatment begins.
- Blood and urine tests check for signs of disease and how well organs are working.
- Imaging tests take pictures of the inside of your body. Imaging tests are used to find and diagnose kidney cancer.
- A biopsy removes a sample of tissue or fluid for testing. Biopsies are not always done before surgery for kidney cancer if the tumor appears to be contained in the kidney. The tumor is usually tested after removal.
- A sample of your tumor may be tested to look for specific DNA (deoxyribonucleic acid) mutations, protein levels, or other molecular features. Some mutations and proteins can be targeted with specific therapies. These tests are more commonly done in those with advanced disease.
- Genetic risk testing might be done to look for gene mutations, inherited from your biological parents, called germline mutations. Some mutations can put you at risk for more than one type of cancer.
- A genetic syndrome that puts someone at risk for developing kidney cancer and possibly other cancers is called hereditary renal cell carcinoma (HRCC).

Those with kidney cancer should be treated at centers experienced in this type of cancer.

3

Kidney cancer staging

Cancer staging is used to reflect prognosis and to guide treatment decisions. It describes the size and location of the tumor and if cancer has spread to lymph nodes, organs, or other parts of the body. This chapter explains kidney cancer stages.

How is kidney cancer staged?

A cancer stage is a way to describe the extent of the cancer at the time you are first diagnosed. The American Joint Committee on Cancer (AJCC) created a staging system to determine how much cancer is in your body, where it is located, and what subtype you have. This is called staging.

Based on testing, your cancer will be assigned a stage. Staging helps to predict prognosis and is needed to make treatment decisions. A prognosis is the course your cancer will likely take. AJCC is just one type of staging system.

Information gathered during staging:

- The extent (size) of the tumor (T): How large is the cancer? Has it grown into nearby areas?
- The spread to nearby lymph nodes (N): Has the cancer spread to nearby lymph nodes? If so, how many? Where?
- The spread (metastasis) to distant sites (M): Has the cancer spread to distant organs such as the lungs or liver?
- Grade of the cancer (G): How much do the cancer cells look like normal cells?

Staging is based on a combination of information to reach a final numbered stage. Often, not all information is available at the initial evaluation. More information can be gathered as treatment begins.

Staging includes:

- **Anatomic –** based on extent of cancer as defined by tumor size (T), lymph node status (N), and distant metastasis (M).
- **Prognostic –** includes anatomic TNM plus tumor grade and other factors such as performance status. The prognostic stage also includes the assumption that you are treated with the standard-of-care approaches.

Prognostic stages are divided into clinical and pathologic. Cancer staging is often done twice, before and after surgery. Staging after surgery provides more specific and accurate details about the size of the cancer, what tissue or organs may be involved, and the presence of cancer in lymph nodes.

Clinical stage

Clinical stage (c) is the rating given before any treatment. It is based on a physical exam, imaging tests, and possible biopsy. An example might look like cN2 or cM1. In kidney cancer, the clinical (before surgery) stage is based mainly on imaging results. These tests are done before any treatment as part of an initial diagnosis. Surgery is needed to know exactly how much cancer is in the body.

Pathologic stage

Pathologic stage (p) or surgical stage is determined by examining tissue removed during surgery. An example might be pN2. If you are given drug therapy before surgery, then the stage might look like ypT3. The pathologic (after surgery) stage is based on information gained after surgery to remove all or part of the kidney and nearby lymph nodes. This gives a more accurate picture of how far the cancer has spread and is used to determine your treatment options after surgery. The removal of tumor tissue is an important part of pathologic staging.

Kidney tumors are measured in centimeters: A baseball is 7 cm, a golf ball is 4 cm, and a pea is 1 cm.

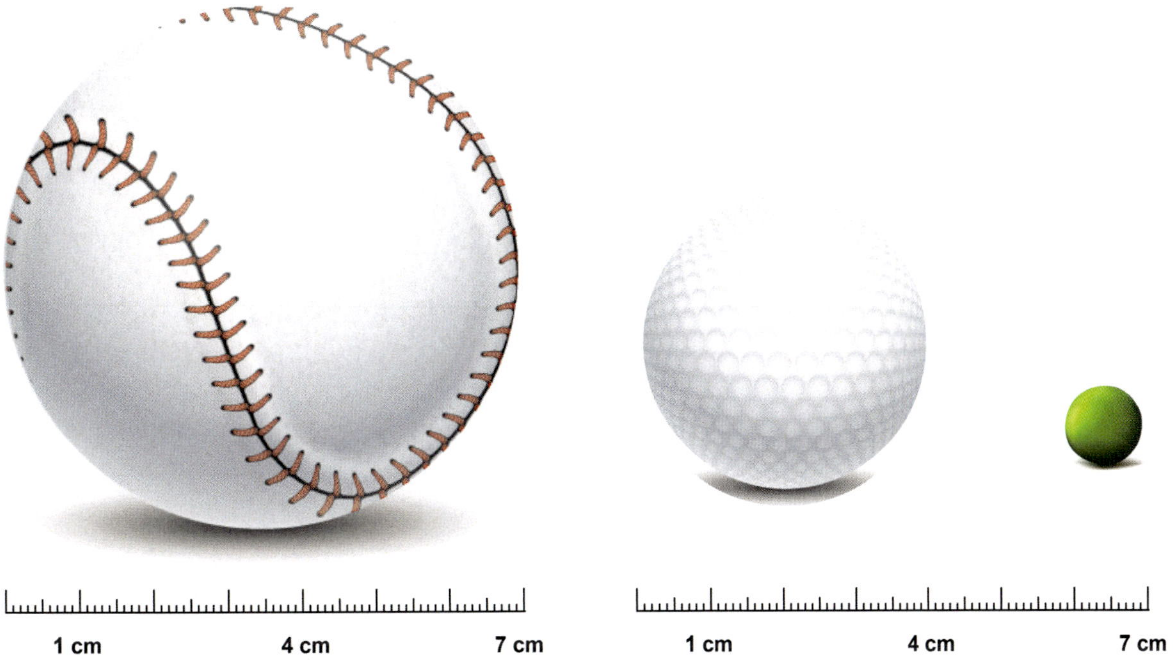

TNM scores

The tumor, node, metastasis (TNM) system is used to stage kidney cancer. In this system, the letters T, N, and M describe different areas of cancer growth. Based on imaging and pathology results, each letter will be assigned a score or number. The higher the number, the larger the tumor or the more the cancer has spread. These scores will be combined to assign the cancer a stage. A TNM example might look like this: T1N0M0 or T1, N0, M0.

- **T is for tumor** – Depth and size of the main (primary) tumor in the kidney
- **N is for node** – If cancer has spread to nearby (regional) lymph nodes
- **M is for metastasis** – If cancer has spread to distant parts of the body

T = Tumor

A tumor can grow outside the kidney and into nearby structures. Kidney tumors are measured in centimeters (cm). A baseball is 7 cm, a golf ball is 4 cm, and a pea is 1 cm. Your kidney is about the size of your fist or about 11 cm by 5 cm.

- **T1** – Tumor is 7 cm or smaller and is limited to the kidney
- **T2** – Tumor is larger than 7 cm and is limited to the kidney
- **T3** – Tumor extends outside the kidney into major veins and tissues, but not into Gerota's fascia
- **T4** – Tumor invades beyond Gerota's fascia and might be in the adrenal gland

N = Regional lymph node

There are hundreds of lymph nodes throughout your body. They work as filters to help fight infection and remove harmful things from your body. Regional lymph nodes are found near the kidney. Regional lymph nodes include renal hilar, caval, and aortic. Cancer found in a regional lymph node is called a lymph node metastasis. This is different than a distant metastasis, which is found far from the main tumor in the kidney.

The removal of lymph nodes is called lymph node or nodal dissection.

- **NX** – Regional lymph nodes cannot be assessed
- **N0** – No regional lymph node metastasis is found
- **N1** – Metastasis in regional lymph node(s) is found

M = Metastasis

Cancer that has spread to distant parts of the body is shown as M1. The most common site for metastasis is the bone, liver, lungs, brain, adrenal glands, and distant lymph nodes.

Grade

Grade describes how abnormal the tumor cells look under a microscope (called histology). Higher-grade cancers tend to grow and spread faster than lower-grade cancers. GX means the grade can't be determined, followed by G1, G2, G3, and G4. G4 is the highest grade for renal cell carcinoma. Tumors with sarcomatoid features are considered G4.

Numbered stages

Numbered stages are based on TNM scores. Stages range from stage 1 to stage 4, with 4 being the most advanced. They might be written as stage I, stage II, stage III, and stage IV.

Other terms might be used instead of numbered cancer stages.

- **Resectable** – Tumor can be removed completely with surgery.
- **Unresectable** – Tumor cannot be removed completely with surgery. The tumor might involve nearby veins and arteries making it unsafe to remove.
- **Locoregional or locally advanced** – This refers to a tumor that has spread to or beyond the blood vessels, tissue, organs, or lymph nodes surrounding the kidney. It may be a stage 3 or 4 tumor, depending on how far outside the kidney the tumor has spread.
- **Metastatic** – Cancer that has spread to other parts of the body, including distant lymph nodes. The most common sites are the lungs, lymph nodes, bones, liver, and the brain. This might be referred to as advanced disease.

Kidney cancer stages

Kidney cancers of the same stage tend to have a similar outcome (prognosis) and are treated in a similar way. In general, earlier cancer stages have better outcomes. Some people will do better than expected. Others will do worse. Factors such as your general health are also very important. **See Guide 2.**

Stage I
T1, N0, M0

The tumor is found only in the kidney and is smaller than 7 cm (T1). Cancer has not spread to nearby lymph nodes (N0) or to other parts of the body (M0).

Stage 2
T2, N0, M0

The tumor is larger than 7 cm and is found only in the kidney (T2). Cancer has not spread to nearby lymph nodes (N0) or to other parts of the body (M0).

Stage 3
T1 or T2, N1, M0

The tumor is found only in the kidney (T1 or T2), but cancer has spread (metastasized) to nearby lymph nodes (N1). This is locally advanced kidney cancer. Cancer has not metastasized to distant sites (M0). The tumor

Guide 2
Kidney cancer stages

Stage 1	• T1, N0, M0
Stage 2	• T2, N0, M0
Stage 3	• T1 or T2, N1, M0 • T3, NX or N1 or N2, M0
Stage 4	• T4, Any N, M0 • Any T, Any N, M1

has not grown into the adrenal gland or beyond Gerota's fascia.

Stage 3
T3, NX or N0 or N1, M0

The tumor has grown outside the kidney into nearby veins and tissues (T3). It has not grown into the adrenal gland or beyond Gerota's fascia. Cancer may or may not be in nearby lymph nodes. If cancer is found in nearby lymph nodes, it is called locally advanced kidney cancer. Cancer has not spread to distant sites (M0).

Stage 4
T4, Any N, M0

The tumor has grown beyond Gerota's fascia and maybe into the adrenal gland (T4). Cancer is found in nearby lymph nodes (N1). Cancer has not metastasized to distant sites in the body (M0). This is locally advanced kidney cancer.

Stage 4 – Metastatic
Any T, Any N, M1

The tumor is any size and may or may not extend beyond the kidney. Cancer may or may not have spread to nearby lymph nodes. Cancer has metastasized to distant parts of the body (M1). This is advanced or metastatic kidney cancer.

Key points

- A cancer stage helps to predict the likely course your cancer will take, called a prognosis. It describes the size and location of the tumor and if cancer has spread to lymph nodes, organs, or other parts of the body.
- Staging is used to make treatment decisions.
- In stage 1 kidney cancer, the tumor is 7 cm or smaller and found only in the kidney.
- In stage 2 kidney cancer, the tumor is larger than 7 cm and found only in the kidney.
- In stage 3 kidney cancer, the tumor has grown outside the kidney into nearby veins and tissues but has not grown into the adrenal gland or beyond Gerota's fascia. Cancer may or may not be in nearby lymph nodes. Cancer has not spread to distant sites.
- In stage 4 kidney cancer, the tumor can be any size. It may have spread outside the kidney. Not all stage 4 kidney cancer is metastatic.

4

Treating kidney cancer

This chapter presents an overview of the possible types of treatment and what to expect. Not everyone will receive the same treatment. Treatment options are based on many factors. Together, you and your care team will choose a treatment plan that is best for you.

Care team

Those with kidney cancer should seek treatment at experienced cancer centers.

Treating cancer takes a team approach. Treatment decisions should involve a multidisciplinary team (MDT). An MDT is a team of health care and psychosocial care professionals from different professional backgrounds who have knowledge (expertise) and experience in your type of cancer. This team is united in the planning and implementing of your treatment. Ask who will coordinate your care.

One or more of the following specialists might be involved in your kidney cancer care:

- **A nephrologist** is an expert in diseases of the kidney.
- **A urologist** is an expert in treating diseases of the urinary system.
- **A urologic oncologist** specializes in diagnosing and treating cancers of the urinary tract. Other types of oncologists include medical, surgical, and radiation.

You know your body better than anyone

Help your care team understand:

- How you feel
- What you need
- What is working and what is not

Keep a list of names and contact information for each member of your team. This will make it easier for you and anyone involved in your care to know whom to contact with questions or concerns.

Get to know your care team and help them get to know you.

Ablation

Ablation is a type of treatment that uses extreme cold or heat, radio waves, microwaves, or chemicals such as ethanol (a type of alcohol) or acetic acid to destroy cancer cells. It can destroy small tumors (typically 3 cm or less) and metastases with little harm to nearby tissue. You might have multiple treatments to destroy the tumor or metastasis. Ablation might be used if you are not healthy enough for surgery or you strongly wish to avoid surgery. A biopsy might be done before or at the time of ablation.

There are many types of ablation used to destroy cancer cells. Those most commonly used to treat a small kidney tumor or an isolated metastasis include:

- **Cryoablation, cryotherapy, or cryosurgery** kills cancer cells by freezing them with a very cold substance.
- **Radiofrequency ablation (RFA)** kills cancer cells by heating them with high-energy radio waves.
- **Microwave ablation** refers to the use of electromagnetic energy to kill cancer cells.

All types of ablation use a special needle, called a probe, which is inserted into the tumor, metastasis, or lesion. With cryotherapy, a medical gas is passed through the probe to cause below-freezing temperatures. This freezes the tumor to destroy it. With RFA, the probe emits radio waves to heat the tumor and destroy it. The probe can be inserted through the skin and guided into place with a CT scan, ultrasound, or other imaging tests. It can also be inserted and guided into place during laparoscopic surgery.

Imaging tests are used to monitor the tumor during treatment to make sure the whole tumor is destroyed (ablated). The probe will be removed when treatment is done.

Active surveillance

Active surveillance happens before treatment.

Surveillance or follow-up care happens after treatment.

Active surveillance closely monitors tumor growth. During this time, you will have imaging tests on a regular basis. You will not have treatment. Treatment will start if the tumor grows or if you are having pain or discomfort. There may be other reasons to start treatment. Ask your care team what might trigger the need for treatment and how often you will have imaging tests.

Active surveillance may be an option for a tumor smaller than 2 cm that has not metastasized or in those with other serious health issues who may not be healthy enough for surgery or other treatments. Age and other health conditions increase the risk of severe side effects and complications from treatment.

Surgery

Surgery is an operation or procedure to remove cancer from the body. Often, surgery is the main or primary treatment to remove the cancer from the kidney. This is only one part of a treatment plan. Surgery can also provide supportive care by easing pain or discomfort. This is called palliative surgery.

When preparing for surgery, you should seek the opinion of an experienced surgeon. The surgeon should be an expert in performing your type of surgery. Hospitals that perform many surgeries often have better results. You can ask for a referral to a hospital or cancer center that has experience in treating your type of cancer.

The removal of the cancer through surgery can be accomplished in different ways depending on the specific circumstances, such as the size and location of the tumor, and if there is cancer in any surrounding organs and tissues. Surgery is based on the safest and best way to remove the cancer.

Open surgery

Open surgery or laparotomy removes tissue through one large surgical cut below your ribs. This approach lets your surgeon directly view and access the tumor in your kidney to remove it. Open surgery may take several hours or longer. After the surgery, you will need to stay in the hospital to recover.

Minimally invasive surgery

Minimally invasive surgery (key-hole surgery) uses a few small incisions. Small tools are inserted through each incision to perform the surgery. One of the tools, called a laparoscope, is a long tube with a video camera at the end. The camera lets your surgeon see your kidney and other tissues inside your abdomen. Other tools are used to remove the tumor. Laparoscopic surgery can also be done using robotic arms to control the surgical tools. This is called robot-assisted laparoscopic surgery.

Tumor resection

The removal of the tumor is called tumor resection. Imaging tests will be ordered to see if your cancer is resectable (can be removed completely by surgery) or unresectable (cannot be removed completely by surgery). Sometimes, imaging tests cannot clearly show one way or the other.

Partial nephrectomy

In a partial nephrectomy, the tumor and tissue immediately surrounding the tumor is removed, leaving behind a still-functioning kidney. The adrenal gland and lymph nodes are also left in your body. A partial nephrectomy might be referred to as nephron-sparing or kidney-sparing surgery since it saves (spares) as much of your kidney as possible. Your kidney can still function even if part of it has been removed. This is a benefit of partial nephrectomy. If you have poor kidney function or are at risk for poor kidney function, this surgery might be an option. It might be an option if you have only one kidney, limited kidney function, or tumors in both kidneys.

Partial nephrectomy is often used for treating kidney cancer when the tumor is small and only in the kidney. A partial nephrectomy can be used to remove larger tumors, but location of the tumor in your kidney and your overall health are considered in any type of surgery. For most small tumors, a partial nephrectomy can remove all the cancer with good long-term results. The surgeon's skill and experience are key factors. Therefore, seek out an experienced surgeon.

Partial nephrectomy is a complex surgery. It is more technically difficult than surgery that removes the whole kidney. A partial nephrectomy should only be done by an expert surgeon who does this type of surgery often.

This surgery should only be done when the entire tumor can be safely removed, leaving the healthy part of the kidney intact.

With any type of surgery, there are health risks and side effects. A side effect is an unhealthy or unpleasant condition caused by treatment. Some possible side effects of a partial nephrectomy include infections, bleeding, pain from the surgical cuts, and urine leaking from the kidney.

Partial nephrectomy

In a partial nephrectomy, the tumor and tissue immediately surrounding the tumor are removed, leaving behind a still-functioning kidney.

https://commons.wikimedia.org/wiki/File:Diagram_showing_before_and_after_a_partial_nephrectomy_CRUK_102.svg

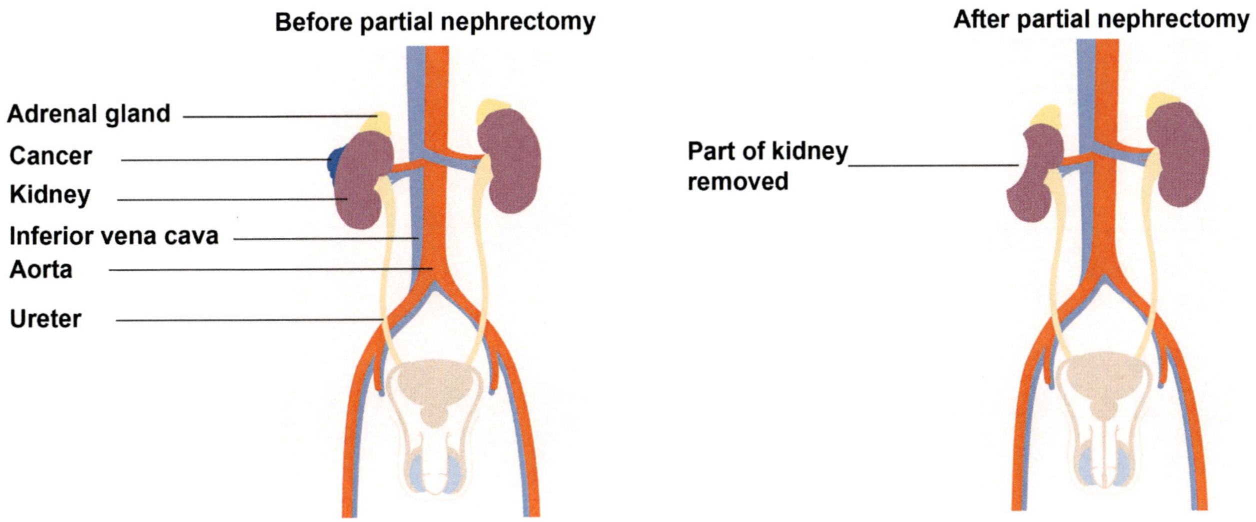

Radical nephrectomy

A radical nephrectomy is surgery that removes the tumor with the whole kidney and the fatty tissue around the kidney. This surgery may also remove the adrenal gland (found on top of the kidney) and nearby lymph nodes. How much tissue is removed depends on the extent of the tumor.

- **Adrenalectomy** removes an adrenal gland. The attached adrenal gland may be removed if it looks abnormal on imaging tests. It may also be removed if the tumor is near the top part of the kidney where the adrenal gland sits.
- **Lymph node dissection** removes nearby lymph nodes. A lymph node dissection is not often done as part of a standard radical nephrectomy. Nearby lymph nodes may be removed if they look enlarged on imaging tests or during surgery.

If the tumor has grown into the renal vein and vena cava, then the veins may be cut open to remove all of the cancer. In rare cases, your heart may need to be stopped for a short time for surgery on the vena cava. While the heart is stopped, a heart-lung machine is used to circulate blood in the body. This is a very difficult and complex procedure. It should only

Radical nephrectomy

In a radical nephrectomy, the tumor with the entire kidney and the fatty tissue around the kidney is removed. This surgery may also remove the adrenal gland on top of the kidney and nearby lymph nodes.

https://commons.wikimedia.org/wiki/File:Diagram_showing_before_and_after_a_radical_nephrectomy_CRUK_104.svg

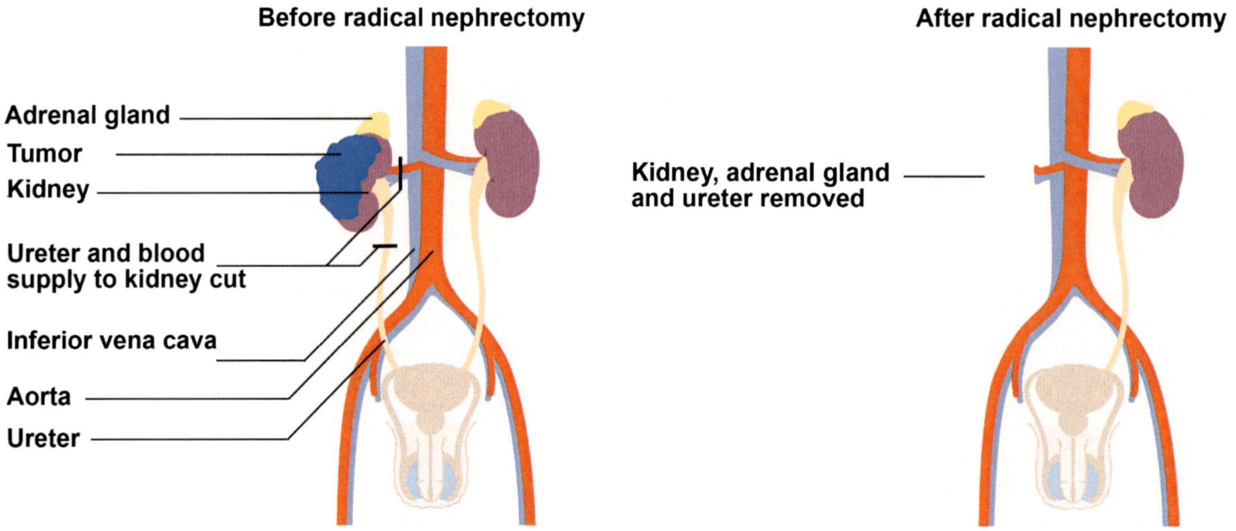

be done by a team of experts who have a lot of experience.

Radical nephrectomy is used to treat kidney cancer when the tumor is large or has invaded nearby tissue. There are many factors that go into deciding which type of surgery might be best for your cancer. Each case is different. Each person is different.

With any type of surgery, there are risks. Some possible side effects of a radical nephrectomy include infection, bleeding, pain, and reduced kidney function. Since the whole kidney is removed, there is an increased risk for chronic kidney disease (CKD). CKD means your remaining kidney can't filter blood the way it should. Kidney function may slowly get worse over a long period of time.

Cytoreductive nephrectomy

A cytoreductive nephrectomy is surgery to remove the primary tumor when you have metastatic kidney cancer. Metastatic cancer has spread from where it first formed to other parts of your body. Cytoreductive surgery is often used to prolong life, reduce pain, or improve quality of life, but not as a cure. Some or all of your kidney might be removed along with the primary tumor in a cytoreductive nephrectomy. Removing the primary tumor may improve how well other treatments work against the remaining cancer and metastases.

A cytoreductive nephrectomy is usually followed by a targeted therapy and/or immunotherapy. It can also be considered in unique cases when the metastases have responded to treatment and there is a large primary tumor. This is sometimes referred to as consolidative surgery. It may also be necessary to consider removal of the tumor if a person develops health issues due to the kidney tumor, such as blood in the urine or severe pain.

Cytoreductive surgery

Not all cancer can be removed from your body with surgery when there are many metastases. Removing some of the cancer metastases, along with the primary tumor, and part or all of your kidney, might help to reduce the amount of cancer in your body, called cancer burden. The goal of cytoreductive surgery is to reduce cancer burden.

Metastasectomy

New tumors that formed far from the primary tumor are called metastases. A metastasectomy is different from a mastectomy (surgery to remove the breast). A metastasectomy is surgery to remove one or more metastases. This surgery may be used when the primary tumor can be completely removed and there is only one metastasis. Not all metastases can be removed by surgery. Location is a key factor. Metastasectomy works best for metastases in the brain, bone, or lung.

A metastasectomy may be done at the same time as surgery to remove the primary tumor, or it may be done during a separate operation. The amount of time needed for the surgery and recovery depends on many factors. Some factors include the size and location of the metastases.

Oligometastases

Oligometastases are a type of metastasis in which cancer cells from the original (primary) tumor travel through the body and form a small number of new tumors (metastatic tumors) in other parts of the body. Treatment for oligometastases or oligometastatic disease includes metastasectomy, radiation therapy, or ablation.

Radiation therapy

Radiation therapy (RT) uses high-energy radiation from x-rays, photons, electrons, and other sources to kill cancer cells and shrink tumors. RT may be used as an ablative therapy instead of surgery, or as a supportive care or palliative care to help ease pain or discomfort caused by cancer.

Stereotactic body radiation therapy (SBRT) is used to treat kidney cancer. In SBRT, a machine outside the body aims radiation beams at the tumor. The goal is to kill or ablate the tumor or metastasis. SBRT can be done with either photons or protons. With this method you will receive high-dose radiation for 1 to 5 treatments. SBRT is very precise, which reduces the chance of damage to nearby tissues.

Systemic therapy

Systemic (drug) therapy works throughout the body. Types include, targeted therapy, immunotherapy, and chemotherapy. Systemic therapy might be used alone or with other therapies. Goals of systemic therapy may be curative or palliative and should be discussed before starting treatment. Your wishes about treatment are important. Make your wishes known.

- **Neoadjuvant or preoperative therapy** is systemic therapy or radiation given before surgery.
- **Perioperative therapy** is systemic therapy given before and after surgery.
- **Adjuvant or postoperative therapy** is systemic therapy or radiation therapy given after surgery.

Guide 3
Systemic therapy examples

Targeted therapy examples	• Axitinib (Inlyta) • Bevacizumab (Avastin) or bevacizumab substitutes (biosimilars) such as Vegzelma, Mvasi, Zirabev, and Alymsys • Cabozantinib (Cabometyx)	• Erlotinib (Tarceva) • Everolimus (Afinitor) • Lenvatinib (Lenvima) • Pazopanib (Votrient) • Sunitinib (Sutent) • Tivozanib (Fotivda)
Immunotherapy examples	• Pembrolizumab (Keytruda) • Nivolumab (Opdivo)	• Ipilimumab (Yervoy) • Avelumab (Bavencio)

- **Palliative therapy** might be the term used for systemic therapy given for advanced or metastatic disease.

For systemic therapy examples, **see Guide 3.**

Targeted therapy

Targeted therapy focuses on specific or unique features of cancer cells. Targeted therapies seek out how cancer cells grow, divide, and move in the body. These drugs stop or inhibit the action of molecules that help cancer cells grow and/or survive. Targeted therapy is used to treat stage 4 (with or without metastases) kidney cancer or cancer that has returned (relapsed). Targeted therapy may have fewer side effects than other types of cancer treatment.

There are 3 types of targeted therapy:

- **Monoclonal antibodies** affect the outside or surface of the cancer cell. A monoclonal antibody (mAb) is a lab-grown protein. There are many kinds of mAbs.
- **Kinase inhibitors** affect the inside of the cancer cell. Kinases move chemicals, called phosphates, from one molecule to another. By transferring phosphates, kinases send signals that tell cells to grow. Kinase inhibitors block these signals.
- **Small molecule inhibitors** bind to target proteins in cells to inhibit their function.

Want to know what drugs are used for?

Look at the last few letters of the drug generic name:

- If it ends in **mab,** it is an **mAb.**
- If it ends in **tinib,** it is a **TKI.**
- If it ends in **limus,** it is an **mTOR.**

Targeted therapy drugs treat kidney cancer in different ways. Some target and block the signals that cause new blood vessels to form. Others block the signals that tell the kidney cancer cells to grow and make more cancer cells. Often, these drugs have more than one target. Targeted therapy drugs are named based on what they target.

In kidney cancer, targeted therapy is used in the following ways:

- **Angiogenesis inhibitors** target blood vessel growth by blocking vascular endothelial growth factor (VEGF) or vascular endothelial growth factor receptors (VEGFR).
- **Hypoxia-inducible factor 2α (HIF-2α) inhibitors** interfere with a cancer cell's ability to sense oxygen and respond to hypoxia (low oxygen states).
- **Mammalian target of rapamycin (mTOR) kinase inhibitors** target cancer cell growth.

Tyrosine kinase inhibitors

Tyrosine kinase inhibitors (TKIs) block the signals that cause kidney cancer to grow and spread. Tyrosine kinases are proteins in cells that are important for many cell functions. This includes sending signals in cells for cell growth, survival, and death. TKIs do not rid the body of cancer. They stop cell growth.

There are many different types of tyrosine kinases. Each TKI works in a slightly different way. Some tyrosine kinases, such as VEGFR, send signals that tell new blood vessels to grow into the tumor. Axitinib (Inlyta) and tivozanib (Fotivda) block VEGFR. Some TKIs target and block more than one type of tyrosine kinase. These are called multi-kinase inhibitors. Many of the multi-kinase inhibitors also block VEGF receptors. Sunitinib (Sutent), pazopanib (Votrient), cabozantinib (Cabometyx), erlotinib (Tarceva), and lenvatinib (Lenvima) are multi-kinase inhibitors.

Hypoxia-inducible factor-2α inhibitors

Hypoxia-inducible factors (HIFs) are transcription factors that sense and respond to low oxygen levels in normal and cancer cells. Belzutifan is a HIF-2α inhibitor that interferes with cancer cell's ability to adapt to low oxygen conditions.

mTOR kinase inhibitors

Mammalian target of rapamycin (mTOR) is a protein in cells that is important for cell growth and survival. mTOR moves chemicals, called phosphates, from one molecule to another. By transferring phosphates, mTOR sends signals that tell cells to grow and divide. An mTOR inhibitor blocks this signal. An example is everolimus (Afinitor). These mTOR kinase inhibitors stop the cell from producing proteins important to RCC and from receiving signals to grow and divide. By blocking the action of mTOR, these drugs slow tumor growth.

Angiogenesis inhibitors

Angiogenesis is the growth of new blood vessels. An angiogenesis inhibitor blocks this growth. Kidney cancer cells are very good at getting new blood vessels to grow into the tumor to feed it. Kidney cancer cells release high amounts of a protein called VEGF.

Bevacizumab (Avastin) and its substitutes are a type of mAb called an angiogenesis inhibitor. Bevacizumab stops VEGF from sending signals that tell new blood vessels to form. This slows or stops blood vessel growth and starves the tumor. Although bevacizumab targets tumor blood vessels, it can also affect normal blood vessels. This can result in side effects. A side effect is a problem caused by treatment.

A biosimilar or substitute might be used in place of bevacizumab. A biosimilar is an almost identical version of a drug made by another company. It is used in the exact same way and at the same dose as bevacizumab. Biosimilars include Vegzelma, Mvasi, Zirabev, and Alymsys. Ask your care team why one therapy might be chosen over another. The reason might be related to tumor mutations, cost, toxicity, or availability. Your wishes are also important.

Immunotherapy

Immunotherapy is a type of systemic treatment that tries to re-activate the immune system against tumor cells. The immune system has many on and off switches. Tumors take advantage of off switches. Immunotherapy can be given alone or with other types of treatment. It is used to treat stage 4 (with or without metastases) kidney cancer or cancer that has returned (relapsed). Sometimes, it is used after surgery to prevent the cancer from coming back.

There are 2 types of immunotherapy used in treating kidney cancer:

- Monoclonal antibody therapy targeting immune checkpoints—also known as immune checkpoint inhibitors (ICIs)
- Cytokine therapy (used only in certain cases)

More information on checkpoint inhibitors and immunotherapy side effects is available at NCCN.org/patientguidelines and on the NCCN Patient Guides for Cancer app.

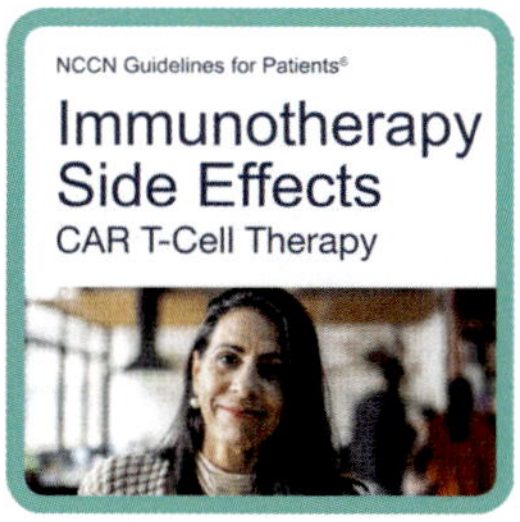

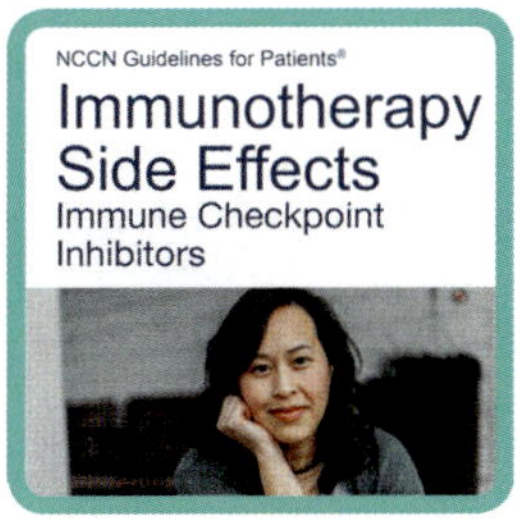

Monoclonal antibody therapy targeting immune checkpoints

Antibody therapy or immune checkpoint inhibitory antibodies are used to help the body fight cancer, infection, or other diseases. Antibodies are proteins made by the immune system that bind to specific markers on cells or tissues. Monoclonal antibodies (mAbs) are a type of antibody made in a lab.

There are 4 immunotherapy mAbs that are approved to treat kidney cancer. All block immune checkpoints and are referred to as immune checkpoint inhibitors (ICIs).

These include:

- Pembrolizumab (Keytruda)
- Nivolumab (Opdivo)
- Ipilimumab (Yervoy)
- Avelumab (Bavencio)

Cytokine therapy

Cytokines are proteins made by our immune system. Some cytokines stimulate the immune system and others slow it down. Interleukin (IL) and interferon are types of cytokine therapy made in a lab that are used only in rare cases for cancer treatment.

Chemotherapy

Chemotherapy is very effective for other types of cancers but is rarely used in the treatment of kidney cancer. It might be an option for treatment of some rare forms of non-clear cell RCC.

Clinical trials

A clinical trial is a type of medical research study. After being developed and tested in a laboratory, potential new ways of treating cancer need to be studied in people. If found to be safe and effective in a clinical trial, a drug, device, or treatment approach may be approved by the U.S. Food and Drug Administration (FDA).

Everyone with cancer should carefully consider all of the treatment options available for their cancer type, including standard treatments and clinical trials. Talk to your doctor about whether a clinical trial may make sense for you.

Phases

Most cancer clinical trials focus on treatment. Treatment trials are done in phases.

- **Phase 1** trials study the dose, safety, and side effects of an investigational drug or treatment approach. They also look for early signs that the drug or approach is helpful.
- **Phase 2** trials study how well the drug or approach works against a specific type of cancer.
- **Phase 3** trials test the drug or approach against a standard treatment. If the results are good, it may be approved by the FDA.
- **Phase 4** trials study the long-term safety and benefit of an FDA-approved treatment.

Who can enroll?

Every clinical trial has rules for joining, called eligibility criteria. The rules may be about age, cancer type and stage, treatment history, lab tests, or general health. These requirements ensure that participants are alike in specific ways and that the trial is as safe as possible for the participants.

Informed consent

Clinical trials are managed by a group of experts called a research team. The research team will review the study with you in detail, including its purpose and the risks and benefits of joining. All of this information is also provided in an informed consent form. Read the form carefully and ask questions before signing it. Take time to discuss with family, friends, or others whom you trust. Keep in mind that you can leave and seek treatment outside of the clinical trial at any time.

Start the conversation

Don't wait for your doctor to bring up clinical trials. Start the conversation and learn about all of your treatment options. If you find a study that you may be eligible for, ask your treatment team if you meet the requirements. If you have already started standard treatment you may not be eligible for certain clinical trials. Try not to be discouraged if you cannot join. New clinical trials are always becoming available.

Frequently asked questions

There are many myths and misconceptions surrounding clinical trials. The possible benefits and risks are not well understood by many with cancer.

Will I get a placebo?

Placebos (inactive versions of real medicines) are almost never used alone in cancer clinical trials. It is common to receive either a placebo with a standard treatment, or a new drug with a standard treatment. You will be informed, verbally and in writing, if a placebo is part of a clinical trial before you enroll.

Do I have to pay to be in a clinical trial?

It depends on the study, your health insurance, and the state in which you live. In general, procedures, drugs, or tests that are considered standard of care will be billed to you or your insurance, whereas those considered research are covered by the trial sponsor. Your treatment team and the research team can help determine if you are responsible for any costs.

Finding a clinical trial

In the United States

NCCN Cancer Centers
NCCN.org/cancercenters

The National Cancer Institute (NCI)
cancer.gov/about-cancer/treatment/clinical-trials/search

Worldwide

The U.S. National Library of Medicine (NLM)
clinicaltrials.gov

Need help finding a clinical trial?

NCI's Cancer Information Service (CIS)
1.800.4.CANCER (1.800.422.6237)
cancer.gov/contact

General supportive care

Supportive care will be specific to your needs. Supportive care is health care given to prevent, reduce, and relieve suffering, and to improve quality of life. Supportive care might include pain relief, palliative care, emotional or spiritual support, financial aid, or family counseling. Tell your care team how you are feeling and about any side effects so they can be managed. Supportive care, best supportive care, and palliative care often mean the same thing.

It is very important to take care of yourself by eating well, drinking plenty of fluids, exercising, and doing things that make you feel energized.

Side effects

All cancer treatments can cause unwanted health issues called side effects. Side effects depend on many factors. These factors include the drug type and dose, length of treatment, and the person. Some side effects may be harmful to your health. Others may just be unpleasant. Treatment can cause several side effects. Some are very serious.

Ask for a complete list of side effects of your treatments. Also, tell your treatment team about any new or worsening symptoms. There may be ways to help you feel better. There are also ways to prevent some side effects. You will be monitored closely for side effects.

Late effects

Late effects are side effects that occur months or years after a disease is diagnosed or after treatment has ended. Late effects may be caused by cancer or cancer treatment. They may include physical, mental, and social health issues, and second cancers. The sooner late effects are treated the better. Ask your care team about what late effects could occur. This will help you know what to look for.

Survivorship

A person is a cancer survivor from the time of diagnosis until the end of life. After treatment, your health will be monitored for side effects of treatment and the return of cancer. This is part of your survivorship care plan. It is important to keep any follow-up doctor visits and imaging test appointments. Seek good routine medical care, including regular doctor visits for preventive care and cancer screening.

A personalized survivorship care plan will contain a summary of possible long-term effects of treatment called late effects and list follow-up tests. Find out how your primary care provider will coordinate with specialists for your follow-up care.

Bone health

Kidney cancer may spread to your bones. This puts your bones at increased risk for injury and disease. Such problems include bone fractures, bone pain, and squeezing (compression) of the spinal cord. High levels of calcium in the blood, called hypercalcemia, may also occur.

You may receive medicine to relieve bone pain and manage low bone density. Some medicines work by slowing or stopping bone breakdown, while others help increase bone thickness. It is recommended that you take calcium and vitamin D with these bone health medicines. Talk to your care team before taking any over-the-counter (OTC) supplements, vitamins, or medicines.

Bone metastases

Bone metastases might be treated with palliative radiation therapy. Medicine to support bone health and to prevent broken bones might also be given.

Distress

Depression, anxiety, and sleeping problems are common and are a normal part of cancer diagnosis. Talk to your care team and with those whom you feel most comfortable about how you are feeling. There are services, people, and medicine that can help you. Support and counseling services are available.

Fatigue

Fatigue is a state of physical or mental tiredness that can be characterized by a lack of energy, motivation, or stamina. Fatigue may be caused by cancer or it may be a side effect of treatment. Let your care team know how you are feeling and if fatigue is getting in the way of doing the things you enjoy. Eating a balanced diet, exercise, yoga, acupuncture, and massage therapy can help. You might be referred to a nutritionist or dietitian to help with fatigue.

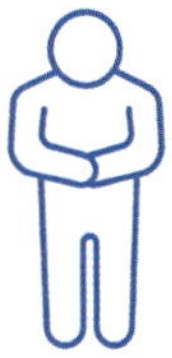

All cancer treatments can cause unwanted health issues called side effects. It is important to tell your care team about all of your side effects so they can be managed.

Supportive care resources

More information on supportive care is available at NCCN.org/patientguidelines and on the NCCN Patient Guides for Cancer app.

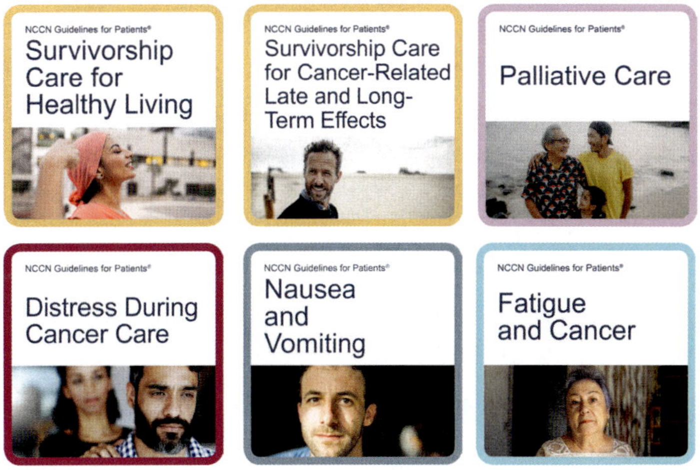

Loss of appetite

Sometimes side effects from cancer or its treatment, and the stress of having cancer might cause you to feel not hungry or sick to your stomach (nauseated). You might have a sore mouth or difficulty swallowing. Healthy eating is important during treatment. It includes eating a balanced diet, eating the right amount of food, and drinking enough fluids. A registered dietitian who is an expert in nutrition and food can help. Speak to your care team if you have trouble eating or maintaining weight.

Nausea and vomiting

Nausea and vomiting are common side effects of treatment. You will be given medicine to prevent nausea and vomiting.

Pain

Tell your care team about any pain or discomfort. You might meet with a palliative care specialist or with a pain specialist to manage pain. Some people may benefit from palliative radiation therapy or ablation therapy to help relieve pain. During this treatment, a radiation beam is focused on the tumor.

Quality of life

Cancer and its treatment can affect your overall well-being or quality of life (QOL). Talk to your care team about how you are feeling.

Warnings about supplements and drug interactions

You might be asked to stop taking or avoid certain herbal supplements when on a systemic therapy. Some supplements can affect the ability of a drug to do its job. This is called a drug interaction.

It is critical to speak with your care team about any supplements you may be taking. Some examples include:

- Turmeric
- Ginkgo biloba
- Green tea extract
- St. John's Wort
- Antioxidants

Certain medicines can also affect the ability of a drug to do its job. Antacids, heart or blood pressure medicine, and antidepressants are just some of the medicines that might interact with a systemic therapy or supportive care medicines given during systemic therapy. Therefore, it is very important to tell your care team about any medicines, vitamins, over-the-counter (OTC) drugs, herbals, or supplements you are taking.

Bring a list with you to every visit.

Key points

- A resectable tumor can be removed with surgery. An unresectable tumor cannot be removed with surgery. Often, surgery is the main or primary treatment for kidney cancer.
- Ablation is a type of treatment that uses extreme cold or heat, radio waves, microwaves, or chemicals to destroy cancer cells.
- Systemic therapy works throughout the body. It includes chemotherapy, targeted therapy, and immunotherapy. Chemotherapy is rarely used in the treatment of kidney cancer
- Radiation therapy (RT) uses high-energy radiation from x-rays, protons, photons, and other sources to kill cancer cells and shrink tumors.
- A clinical trial is a type of research that studies a treatment to see how safe it is and how well it works.
- Supportive care is health care that relieves symptoms caused by cancer or its treatment and improves quality of life. Supportive care is always given.
- All cancer treatments can cause unwanted health issues called side effects. It is important for you to tell your care team about all your side effects so they can be managed.

5

Stages 1, 2, and 3

Kidney cancer confined to the kidney is usually treated with surgery. Depending on the stage, active surveillance or ablation might be options. After treatment, you will have follow-up care. Together, you and your care team will choose a treatment plan that is best for you.

Usually, localized kidney cancer is treated with surgery.

- **In a partial nephrectomy,** the tumor and tissue immediately surrounding the tumor are removed, leaving behind a still-functioning kidney.
- **In a radical nephrectomy,** the tumor with the whole kidney and the fatty tissue around the kidney are removed. The adrenal gland and nearby lymph nodes may also be removed.

Depending on the cancer stage, active surveillance or ablation might be an option. After treatment, you will have follow-up care. A follow-up plan will be based on your situation. Treatment options for stages 1, 2, and 3 can be found in **Guide 4.**

Stage 1 (T1a)

In stage 1 (T1a) cancer, the tumor is 4 cm or smaller and found only in the kidney. A partial nephrectomy is the preferred treatment option. Ablation and active surveillance are also options. A radical nephrectomy would be used only in some cases.

During active surveillance

Those with tumors smaller than 2 cm in size are ideal candidates for active surveillance due to the low likelihood that the tumor will spread during observation. This may also be a good option for smaller tumors that are primarily cystic (fluid filled).

Active surveillance includes:

- Physical exam and health history every year
- Blood and urine tests, as needed
- Abdominal CT or MRI with and without contrast within 6 months of starting surveillance, then CT, MRI, or ultrasound (US) at least every year
- A chest x-ray or CT baseline and annual as needed to look for lung metastases
- Other tests as needed based on symptoms, side effects, and other health concerns

Stage 1 (T1b)

In stage 1b cancer, the tumor is larger than 4 cm but not larger than 7 cm in size and found only in the kidney. Treatment options include a partial or radical nephrectomy. Active surveillance or ablation might be an option in certain cases.

Stage 2

In stage 2 cancer, the tumor is larger than 7 cm and found only in the kidney. Treatment is a partial or radical nephrectomy. Treatment surgery is called adjuvant therapy. Adjuvant therapy might include surveillance or pembrolizumab.

Stage 3

In stage 3 kidney cancer, the tumor has grown outside the kidney into nearby veins and tissues, but has not grown into the adrenal gland or beyond Gerota's fascia. Cancer has not spread to distant sites. Stage 3 kidney cancer is treated with a radical nephrectomy. A partial nephrectomy might be an option in certain cases.

Treatment after surgery is called adjuvant therapy. For stage 3 RCC, adjuvant therapy includes pembrolizumab, surveillance, or a clinical trial.

Guide 4
Primary treatment options based on cancer stage

Stage 1 (T1a)	• Partial nephrectomy (preferred) • Ablation • Active surveillance • Radical nephrectomy (in some cases)	➡	Followed by surveillance
Stage 1 (T1b)	• Partial nephrectomy • Radical nephrectomy • Active surveillance (in some cases) • Ablation (in some cases)	➡	Followed by surveillance
Stage 2	• Partial nephrectomy • Radical nephrectomy, as needed	➡	Followed by • Surveillance • Adjuvant pembrolizumab (for grade 4 clear cell tumors with or without sarcomatoid features)
Stage 3	• Radical nephrectomy • Partial nephrectomy, as needed	➡	Followed by • If clear cell, then adjuvant pembrolizumab or surveillance • If non-clear cell, then surveillance or clinical trial

Follow-up care

Follow-up care includes regular physical exams, health history, and blood, urine, and imaging tests. Other tests might be ordered if you are having any symptoms or as needed.

After 5 years

Long-term follow-up care will include a physical exam and health history. Other tests including imaging, blood, and urine tests may be ordered if you are having any symptoms. The goal of care is to monitor kidney function and watch for cancer return or metastatic disease. Those with hereditary RCC will likely need lifelong follow-up care.

Palliative care is appropriate for anyone, regardless of age, cancer stage, or the need for other therapies. It focuses on physical, emotional, social, and spiritual needs that affect quality of life (QOL).

Seek out support groups at your local hospital, through social media, or through resources listed in the back of this book. Look to friends, relatives, neighbors, and peers for social support.

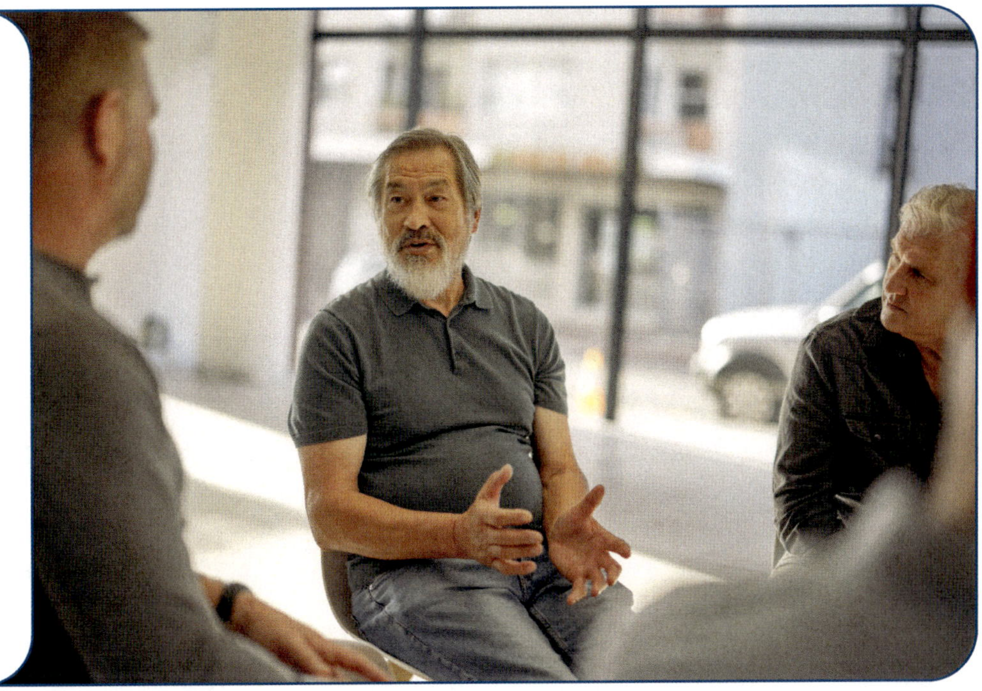

Key points

- In stage 1a cancer, the tumor is 4 cm or smaller and found only in the kidney.
- In stage 1b cancer, the tumor is larger than 4 cm but not larger than 7 cm in size and found only in the kidney.
- In stage 2 kidney cancer, the tumor is larger than 7 cm and found only in the kidney. In stage 2A, the tumor is 7 cm to 10 cm in diameter. In stage 2B the tumor is larger than 10 cm.
- In stage 3 kidney cancer, the tumor has grown outside the kidney into nearby veins and tissues, but has not grown into the adrenal gland or beyond Gerota's fascia. Cancer has not spread to distant sites.
- For high-grade stage 2 RCC or stage 3 RCC, treatment after surgery (called adjuvant therapy) will be given.
- Follow-up care will include a physical exam and health history, along with imaging, blood, and urine tests. The goal of care is to monitor kidney function and watch for cancer return or metastatic disease. Those with hereditary RCC will likely need lifelong follow-up care.

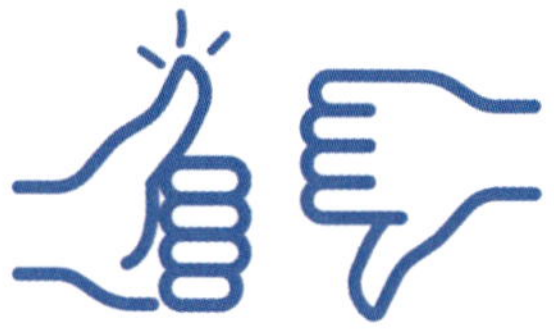

Let us know what you think!

Please take a moment to complete an online survey about the NCCN Guidelines for Patients.

NCCN.org/patients/response

6

Stage 4 and relapse

This chapter discusses treatment options for stage 4 and relapsed disease. Relapse is the return of cancer. In metastatic disease, cancer has spread to distant sites in the body. Not all stage 4 kidney cancers are metastatic. Together, you and your care team will choose a treatment plan that is best for you.

Stage 4

In stage 4 kidney cancer, the tumor has grown outside the kidney and Gerota's fascia and/or has spread to a distant site. Kidney cancer that has spread to a distant site is called metastatic renal cell carcinoma (mRCC). Not all stage 4 kidney cancer is metastatic. Non-metastatic stage 4 kidney cancer is called advanced RCC.

Treatment for stage 4 kidney cancer is based on your symptoms. If there are metastases, treatment will be based on the number and location of metastases. A biopsy might be taken of one or more of these metastases.

Surgery

If surgery is an option, then you might have a nephrectomy followed by pembrolizumab or surveillance. A clinical trial is an option for non-clear cell RCC.

For metastatic disease, you might have cytoreductive nephrectomy. In cytoreductive nephrectomy, all or part of the kidney with the tumor is removed. When there are many metastases, it is not always possible to remove them all. Removing the primary tumor may improve how well other treatments work against the remaining cancer and metastases. A cytoreductive nephrectomy is usually followed by targeted therapy and/or immunotherapy. Systemic therapy options are the same used to treat relapse disease found in the section below.

Systemic therapy

If you did not have surgery, then a sample of the tumor (biopsy) will be taken and tested to determine if the cancer is a clear cell or non-clear cell subtype. Subtype affects treatment options, which can be found in the next section on Relapse.

Relapse

Recurrence or relapse is the return of cancer. Prognostic risk factors help estimate the risk of cancer recurrence and survival. These factors include overall performance status (activity level), blood counts, blood calcium and LDH levels, and the time from primary surgery to metastatic disease.

- If a person with metastatic RCC has no risk factors, they are considered favorable risk.
- If a person has 1 to 2 risk factors, they are considered intermediate risk.
- Those with 3 or more risk factors are considered poor risk.

Before starting treatment, a sample of your tumor (biopsy) will be tested to determine the subtype of RCC. When kidney cancer cells form new tumors in other parts of the body, it is referred to as metastatic disease. A biopsy might be taken of one or more of these metastases.

Systemic therapy options are based on whether you have had any systemic therapy before (as adjuvant therapy) and your overall health, including other medical conditions.

Clear cell

Treatment options include:

- Clinical trial
- First-line systemic therapy
- For oligometastatic disease, metastasectomy, radiation therapy (SBRT), or ablation
- Metastasectomy with complete resection of disease, followed by adjuvant pembrolizumab within 1 year of nephrectomy and best supportive care

First-line therapies are the initial systemic treatments given for metastatic RCC. Options are based on whether you have had any systemic therapy before in the adjuvant setting and your overall health, including other medical conditions and prognostic risk factors. First line-systemic therapy options for clear cell RCC can be found in **Guide 5.**

Guide 5
First-line systemic therapy options: Clear cell RCC

Preferred	Favorable risk: • Axitinib with pembrolizumab • Cabozantinib with nivolumab • Lenvatinib with pembrolizumab • Ipilimumab with nivolumab	Intermediate or poor risk: • Axitinib with pembrolizumab • Cabozantinib with nivolumab • Ipilimumab with nivolumab • Lenvatinib with pembrolizumab • Cabozantinib
Other recommended	Favorable risk: • Axitinib with avelumab • Cabozantinib • Pazopanib • Sunitinib	Intermediate or poor risk: • Axitinib with avelumab • Pazopanib • Sunitinib
Used in some cases	Favorable risk: • Active surveillance • Axitinib	Intermediate or poor risk: • Axitinib

Non-clear cell

Treatment options for non-clear cell RCC include:

- Clinical trial (preferred)
- Systemic therapy
- For oligometastatic disease, metastasectomy, radiation therapy (SBRT), or ablation
- Best supportive care

Best supportive care is used to relieve symptoms caused by cancer or cancer treatment and improve quality of life.

First-line systemic therapy options for non-clear cell RCC can be found in **Guide 6.**

Follow-up care

Follow-up tests are used to monitor your health. It will be based on your treatment, side effects, health issues, symptoms, and subtype of kidney cancer. Follow-up care will include blood and imaging tests. A baseline test is a starting point to which future tests are compared. After the baseline test, ongoing imaging tests are used to show if the cancer grows or shrinks over time.

Disease progression

When cancer grows or spreads, it is called disease progression. When first-line systemic therapy doesn't stop the growth or spread of cancer, then more lines of therapy might be given. Treatment is based on the type of systemic therapy you had before (as adjuvant therapy) and your overall health, including other medical conditions.

Guide 6
Systemic therapy options: Non-clear cell RCC

Preferred	• Clinical trial • Cabozantinib	• Cabozantinib with nivolumab • Lenvatinib with pembrolizumab
Other recommended	• Erlotinib with bevacizumab for some people with advanced papillary RCC including hereditary leiomyomatosis and renal cell cancer (HLRCC)-associated RCC	• Everolimus with lenvatinib • Nivolumab • Pembrolizumab • Sunitinib
Used in some cases	• Axitinib • Everolimus with bevacizumab	• Everolimus • Ipilimumab with nivolumab

Treatment options include:

- Clinical trial (preferred)
- Systemic therapy
- For oligometastatic disease, metastasectomy, radiation therapy (SBRT), or ablation
- Best supportive care

Supportive care is given to relieve the symptoms of cancer or side effects of cancer treatment. Best supportive care aims to improve quality of life and relieve any discomfort you may have. It may include surgery, systemic, or other treatments. Radiation therapy may be used to relieve pain from cancer that has spread to your bones or brain. Drugs that strengthen your bones may also help with pain and other problems caused by bone metastases.

Clear cell

Next-line or subsequent therapies are those given after first-line therapies. You will have a different drug therapy than before. Next-line systemic therapy options in those with clear cell RCC can be found in **Guide 7.**

Non-clear cell

Next-line systemic therapy for non-clear cell RCC can be found in **Guide 6.**

Guide 7
Next-line systemic therapy options: Clear cell RCC

Recommended	No prior immunotherapy: • Axitinib with pembrolizumab • Cabozantinib • Cabozantinib with nivolumab • Everolimus with lenvatinib • Ipilimumab with nivolumab • Lenvatinib with pembrolizumab • Nivolumab	Prior immunotherapy: • Axitinib • Belzutifan • Cabozantinib • Everolimus with lenvatinib • Tivozanib
Used in some cases	No prior immunotherapy: • Axitinib • Everolimus • Pazopanib • Sunitinib • Tivozanib • Belzutifan • Bevacizumab	Prior immunotherapy: • Axitinib with pembrolizumab • Cabozantinib with nivolumab • Everolimus • Ipilimumab with nivolumab • Lenvatinib with pembrolizumab • Pazopanib • Sunitinib • Bevacizumab

Key points

- In stage 4 kidney cancer, the tumor has grown outside the kidney and Gerota's fascia and/or has spread to a distant site.
- Kidney cancer that has spread to a distant site is called metastatic RCC (mRCC). Not all stage 4 kidney cancer is metastatic. Non-metastatic stage 4 kidney cancer is called advanced RCC.
- Treatment is based on your symptoms and clear cell or non-clear cell subtype. If there are metastases, treatment will be based on the number and location of metastases.
- Follow-up testing will monitor for relapse or disease progression.
- Prognostic risk factors help estimate the risk of cancer recurrence and survival. These factors include overall performance status (activity level), blood counts, blood calcium and LDH levels, and the time from primary surgery to metastatic disease.
- Supportive care is given to relieve the symptoms of cancer or side effects of cancer treatment.
- Best supportive care aims to improve quality of life and relieve any discomfort you may have. It may include radiation therapy, surgery, systemic therapy, or other treatments.

Standard of care is the best-known way to treat a particular disease based on past clinical trials. There may be more than one treatment regimen that is considered standard of care. Ask your care team what treatment options are available and if a clinical trial might be right for you.

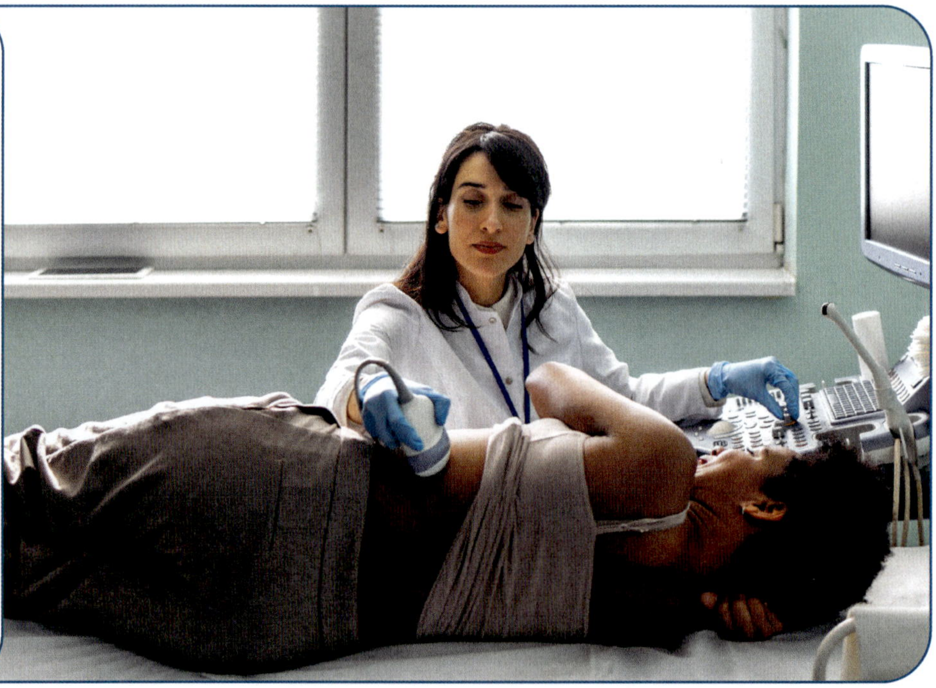

7

Hereditary RCC

Certain genetic conditions can put you at risk for developing kidney cancer. This is called hereditary renal cell carcinoma (HRCC). Most people with confirmed HRCC are treated with kidney-sparing surgery. Other options might include ablation or systemic therapy, depending on the type of HRCC.

Overview

Kidney cancer often occurs for unknown reasons. Some people have genetic health conditions that increase the risk for developing kidney cancer. This is called hereditary renal cell carcinoma (HRCC).

HRCC types include:

- Von Hippel-Lindau (VHL) disease
- Hereditary papillary renal carcinoma (HPRC)
- Birt-Hogg-Dubé syndrome (BHDS)
- Tuberous sclerosis complex (TSC)
- Hereditary leiomyomatosis and renal cell carcinoma (HLRCC)
- *BAP1* tumor predisposition syndrome (*BAP1*-TPDS)
- Hereditary paraganglioma/pheochromocytoma (PGL/PCC) syndrome

HRCC is the result of mutations in DNA passed down from biological parent to child through genes. Those with HRCC have a higher risk for kidney cancer and possibly other cancer not related to the kidney. HRCC accounts for only a small portion of kidney cancer cases.

For more information on HRCC, see **Guide 8.**

Treatment

Most with confirmed HRCC are treated with kidney-sparing surgery (partial nephrectomy). Other options might include ablation or systemic therapy, depending on the type of HRCC. If possible, seek treatment with a doctor or hospital that is experienced in your type of HRCC.

BAP1-TPDS

BAP1 tumor predisposition syndrome *(BAP1*-TPDS) is caused by mutations in the *BAP1* gene and is associated with increased risks for uveal and skin melanoma, mesothelioma, and RCC. There are no specific treatment guidelines for this syndrome.

Birt-Hogg-Dubé syndrome

Birt-Hogg-Dubé syndrome (BHDS) is associated with multiple non-cancerous (benign) skin tumors, lung cysts, and an increased risk of kidney lesions (cysts, benign tumors, and kidney cancer). When possible, a partial nephrectomy is the treatment of choice for kidney tumors. A person may have multiple tumors during their lifetime and, therefore, might have more than one surgery. This will be taken into consideration. Ablation may be an option if surgery is not possible or the best choice for your situation.

Hereditary leiomyomatosis and RCC

Hereditary leiomyomatosis and renal cell carcinoma (HLRCC) increases the risk for developing multiple smooth muscle tumors (leiomyomas) in the skin and uterus (fibroids), as well as an aggressive form of papillary kidney cancer. Since HLRCC tumors can be aggressive, surveillance is not recommended. A total radical nephrectomy should be considered. There are no specific FDA-approved therapies for HLRCC. Treatment with erlotinib plus bevacizumab (or its biosimilar) has shown benefit in those with metastatic RCC from HLRCC.

Guide 8
Hereditary RCC types

Syndrome	Mutation	Common RCC type
von Hippel-Lindau (VHL)	*VHL* gene	Clear cell
Hereditary papillary renal carcinoma (HPRC)	*MET* gene	Papillary
Birt-Hogg-Dubé syndrome (BHDS)	*FLCN* gene	Chromophobe, hybrid oncocytic tumors, clear cell, oncocytomas, angiomyolipomas, papillary RCC
Tuberous sclerosis complex (TSC)	*TSC1* and *TSC2* genes	Angiomyolipoma (and other PEComas), renal cysts, eosinophilic solid and cystic RCC, RCC with fibromyomatous stroma, eosinophilic vacuolated tumor, low-grade oncocytic tumor, clear cell
Hereditary leiomyomatosis and renal cell carcinoma (HLRCC)	*FH* gene	HLRCC-associated RCC or FH-deficient RCC
***BAP1* tumor predisposition syndrome (*BAP1*-TPDS)**	*BAP1* gene	Clear cell
Hereditary paraganglioma/ pheochromocytoma (PGL/PCC) syndrome	*SDHA*, *SDHB*, *SDHC*, and *SDHD* genes	SDH-deficient RCC

Hereditary papillary renal carcinoma

Hereditary papillary renal carcinoma (HPRC) increases the risk of a type of kidney cancer known as papillary type 1 kidney cancer.

Mutations in the *MET* gene cause abnormal cells to grow and spread in the body. Those with HPRC have an increased risk of multiple kidney tumors in one or both kidneys (also called bilateral kidney tumors). Currently, surgery is the primary method when a localized tumor reaches greater than 3 cm in size. When possible, a partial nephrectomy is the treatment of choice. A person may have multiple tumors during their lifetime and, therefore, might have more than one surgery. This will be taken into consideration when planning treatment. Ablation is also an option.

Hereditary paraganglioma-pheochromocytoma syndrome

Hereditary paraganglioma-pheochromocytoma (PGL/PCC) syndromes are characterized by paragangliomas and pheochromocytomas.

- **Paragangliomas** are tumors that arise from neuroendocrine tissues found along the spine from the base of the skull to the pelvis.
- **Pheochromocytomas** are a type of paraganglioma that is confined to the adrenal gland, a small hormone-producing organ located on top of each kidney.

Paragangliomas and pheochromocytomas can occur in individuals with other inherited disorders, such as von Hippel-Lindau syndrome.

Malignant tumors without aggressive features and early stage should undergo surgical resection. A partial nephrectomy can be considered. For larger tumors and those with aggressive features (such as high grade or sarcomatoid), radical nephrectomy should be considered.

Tuberous sclerosis complex

Tuberous sclerosis complex (TSC) is characterized by the growth of numerous noncancerous (benign) tumors in many parts of the body. These tumors can occur in the skin, brain, kidneys, and other organs. Almost everyone with TSC has skin abnormalities. Kidney tumors are common in those with TSC. Partial nephrectomy is the treatment of choice for malignant (cancerous) kidney tumors, when possible. Ablation is also an option.

Renal angiomyolipoma is a benign lesion associated with TSC and is managed separately.

Everolimus is an FDA-approved therapy for asymptomatic, growing angiomyolipoma measuring larger than 3 cm in diameter.

Von Hippel-Lindau

In von Hippel-Lindau (VHL) disease, a mutation in the *VHL* gene causes tumors and cysts to grow in certain areas of the body and increases the chance of developing kidney cancer and other cancers. The goal of treatment is to intervene at a time when there will be the most benefit and to limit the chance of developing metastatic disease. You should be referred to a hospital or cancer center with surgical expertise in complex partial nephrectomies and management of VHL.

Surgery has been the primary method when a localized tumor reaches greater than 3 cm in size. A person may have multiple tumors during their lifetime and, therefore, might have more than one surgery. This will be taken into consideration when planning treatment. Ablation may be an option if surgery is not possible. Belzutifan (Welireg) can be used for the treatment of VHL disease-related renal cell carcinomas, hemangioblastomas, and pancreatic neuroendocrine tumors and can be considered as an alternative to surgery if surgery can wait. Pazopanib might be an option in some cases.

Key points

- Kidney cancer related to an inherited syndrome is called hereditary renal cell carcinoma (HRCC). There are several conditions that cause HRCC.
- Those who have HRCC should see their doctors often, especially if they have already been diagnosed with RCC. Regular imaging tests will look for new kidney tumors.
- Most with confirmed HRCC are treated with kidney-sparing surgery (partial nephrectomy). Other options might include ablation or systemic therapy, depending on the type of HRCC. Seek treatment with a doctor or hospital that is experienced in your type of HRCC.

Your preferences about treatment are always important. If you have any religious or personal beliefs about certain kinds of treatment, share them with your care team and make your wishes known.

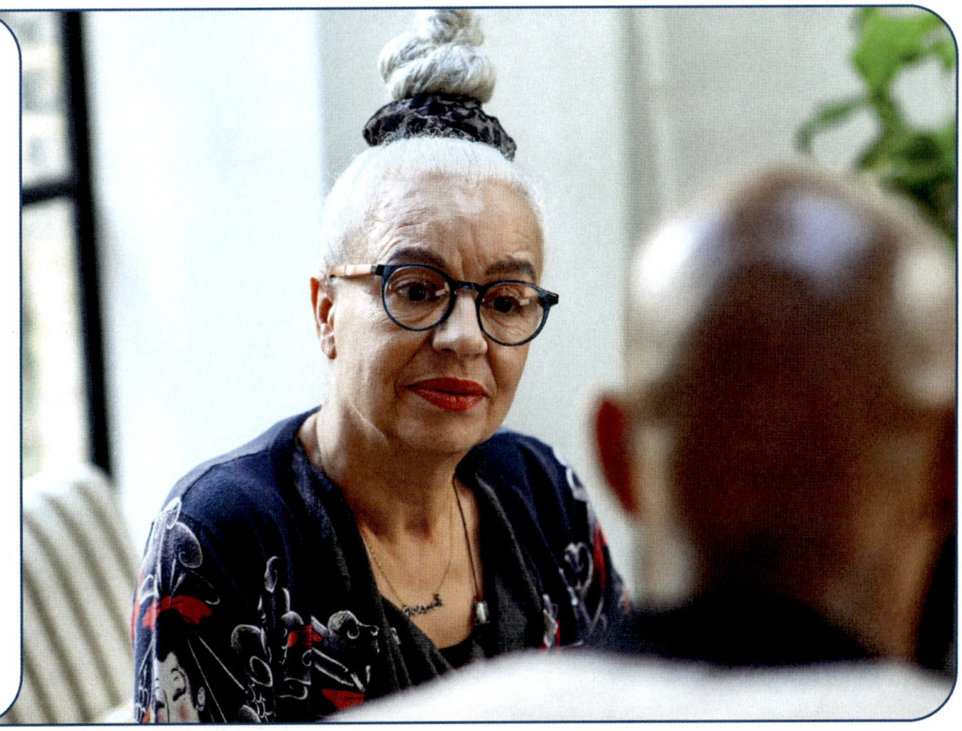

8
Making treatment decisions

It's important to be comfortable with the cancer treatment you choose. This choice starts with having an open and honest conversation with your care team.

It's your choice

In shared decision-making, you and your care team share information, discuss the options, and agree on a treatment plan. It starts with an open and honest conversation between you and your care team.

Treatment decisions are very personal. What is important to you may not be important to someone else. Some things that may play a role in your decision-making:

- What you want and how that might differ from what others want
- Your religious and spiritual beliefs
- Your feelings about certain treatments
- Your feelings about pain or side effects
- Cost of treatment, travel to treatment centers, and time away from school, work, or family
- Quality of life and length of life
- How active you are and the activities that are important to you

Think about what you want from treatment. Discuss openly the risks and benefits of specific treatments and procedures. Weigh options and share concerns with your care team. If you take the time to build a relationship with your care team, it will help you feel supported when considering options and making treatment decisions.

Second opinion

It is normal to want to start treatment as soon as possible. While cancer can't be ignored, there is time to have another doctor review your test results and suggest a treatment plan. This is called getting a second opinion, and it's a normal part of cancer care. Even doctors get second opinions!

Things you can do to prepare:

- Check with your insurance company about its rules on second opinions. There may be out-of-pocket costs to see doctors who are not part of your insurance plan.
- Make plans to have copies of all your records sent to the doctor you will see for your second opinion.

Support groups

Many people diagnosed with cancer find support groups to be helpful. Support groups often include people at different stages of treatment. Some people may be newly diagnosed, while others may be finished with treatment. If your hospital or community doesn't have support groups for people with cancer, check out the websites listed in this book.

Questions to ask

Possible questions to ask your care team are listed on the following pages. Feel free to use these questions or come up with your own. Be clear about your goals for treatment and find out what to expect from treatment.

Questions about testing and diagnosis

1. What type and stage of cancer do I have? What does this mean in terms of my prognosis and treatment options?
2. Is there a cancer center or hospital nearby that specializes in this type of cancer?
3. Will treatment start before the test results are in?
4. What tests will I have?
5. Will my insurance pay for this test?
6. How soon will I know the test results and who will explain them to me?
7. What are the next steps?
8. Is my cancer resectable or unresectable? What does this mean?
9. Is the cancer early stage, locally advanced, or metastatic?
10. Is the cancer in areas like my liver, lungs, or bone?

Questions about your care team's experience

1. What is your experience treating this type of cancer?
2. What is the experience of those on your team?
3. What types of cancer do you treat?
4. I would like to get a second opinion. Is there someone you recommend?
5. How many people like me (of the same age, gender, race) have you treated?
6. Will you be consulting with experts to discuss my care? Whom will you consult?
7. How many procedures like the one you're suggesting have you done?
8. Is this treatment a major part of your practice?
9. What types of complications are possible?
10. Who will manage my day-to-day care?

Questions about options

1. Which option is proven to work best for my cancer, age, overall health, and other factors?
2. What will happen if I do nothing?
3. Am I a candidate for a clinical trial?
4. Can I join a clinical trial at any time?
5. What if I am pregnant or am planning to get pregnant soon?
6. Can I stop treatment at any time? What will happen if I stop treatment?
7. What are my options if treatment doesn't work as expected?
8. What decisions must be made today? Is there a social worker or someone who can help me decide about treatment?
9. Can I go to one hospital for surgery and a different center for radiation therapy?

Questions about treatment

1. Which treatment(s) do you recommend and why?
2. Does this treatment offer a cure? If not, how well can treatment stop the cancer from growing?
3. Does the order of treatment matter?
4. When will I start treatment and how long will treatment likely take?
5. What should I expect from treatment?
6. What will you do to make me comfortable during treatment?
7. How much will my insurance pay for treatment?
8. Are there programs to help me pay for treatment?
9. What are the chances my cancer will return?

Questions about surgery

1. How much of the tumor and kidney will be removed?
2. What other organs or tissues might be removed during surgery?
3. Does my cancer involve any veins or arteries and how might this affect surgery?
4. Will I have or need more than one surgery?
5. Will the incision be on my front, side, or back?
6. How long will recovery take and what should I expect?
7. How much pain will I be in and what will be done to manage my pain?
8. How will surgery affect kidney function, blood pressure, or my health in general?
9. Am I at risk for chronic kidney disease (CKD)?
10. What treatment will I have before, during, or after surgery?

Questions about radiation therapy

1. What type of radiation therapy (RT) will I have?
2. What will you target?
3. What is the goal of this radiation treatment?
4. Will RT be used with other therapies?
5. How many treatment sessions will I require?
6. Do you offer this type of radiation here? If not, can you refer me to someone who does?
7. What side effects can I expect from RT?
8. Will I be given medicine to help me relax during RT?
9. What should I wear?

Questions about clinical trials

1. What clinical trials are available for my grade and stage of cancer?
2. What are the treatments used in the clinical trial?
3. What does the treatment do?
4. Has the treatment been used before? Has it been used for other types of cancer?
5. What are the risks and benefits of this treatment?
6. What side effects should I expect? How will the side effects be controlled?
7. How long will I be in the clinical trial?
8. Will I be able to get other treatments if this doesn't work?
9. How will you know the treatment is working?
10. Will the clinical trial cost me anything? If so, how much?

Questions about side effects

1. What are the side effects of this treatment?
2. How are these side effects treated?
3. How long will these side effects last?
4. Do any side effects lessen or worsen in severity over time?
5. What side effects are expected and which are life threatening?
6. When should I call my care team?
7. What should I do for an issue on weekends and other non-office hours?
8. What medicines can I take to prevent or relieve side effects?
9. Will you stop treatment or change treatment if there are side effects? What do you look for?
10. What can I do to help lessen pain or other side effects?

Questions about resources and support

1. Who can I talk to about help with housing, food, and other basic needs?
2. What help is available for transportation, childcare, and home care?
3. How much will I have to pay for treatment?
4. What help is available to pay for medicines and other treatment?
5. What other services are available to me and my caregivers?
6. How can I connect with others and build a support system?
7. How can I find in-person or online support?
8. Who can help me with my concerns about missing work or school?
9. Who can I talk to if I don't feel safe at home, at work, or in my neighborhood?
10. How can I get help to stop smoking or vaping?

Notes

Resources

Cancer*Care*
Cancercare.org

Cancer Hope Network
cancerhopenetwork.org

Imerman Angels
imermanangels.org

International Kidney Cancer Coalition
ikcc.org

KidneyCAN
kidneycan.org

Kidney Cancer Association
kidneycancer.org

MedlinePlus
medlineplus.gov

National Cancer Institute (NCI)
cancer.gov/types/kidney

National Coalition for Cancer Survivorship
canceradvocacy.org

Triage Cancer
triagecancer.org

We want your feedback!

Our goal is to provide helpful and easy-to-understand information on cancer.

Take our survey to let us know what we got right and what we could do better.

NCCN.org/patients/feedback

Words to know

active surveillance
Frequent and ongoing testing to watch for cancer growth without giving active treatment.

adrenal gland
A small organ on top of each kidney that makes hormones.

adrenalectomy
Surgery that removes the adrenal gland. The adrenal gland might be removed in a radical nephrectomy.

angiogenesis
The growth of new blood vessels.

angiogenesis inhibitor
A drug that blocks the growth of new blood vessels that feed cancer cells.

baseline
A starting point to which future test results are compared.

best supportive care
Treatment to improve quality of life and relieve discomfort. Also called palliative care or supportive care.

biopsy
The removal of a sample of tissue for testing.

biosimilar
A drug that is very much like one that has been approved by the U.S. Food and Drug Administration (FDA). It must be used in the exact same way and at the same dose as the other drug.

bone scan
An imaging test that uses radioactive material to check for cancer or damage in bones.

cancer burden
The amount or extent of cancer in the body.

cancer stage
A rating of the growth and spread of cancer.

carcinoma
A cancer of cells that line the inner or outer surfaces of the body.

chromophobe RCC (cRCC)
Subtype of RCC (renal cell carcinoma) based on how the cancer cells look when viewed with a microscope.

clear cell RCC (ccRCC)
The most common subtype of RCC (renal cell carcinoma) based on how the cancer cells look when viewed with a microscope.

clinical stage (c)
Rating the extent of a tumor based on tests before treatment is started.

clinical trial
Research on a test or treatment to assess its safety or how well it works.

collecting duct RCC (cdRCC)
Subtype of renal cell carcinoma (RCC) based on how the cancer cells look when viewed with a microscope.

computed tomography (CT)
A test that combines many x-rays to make pictures of the inside of the body.

contrast
A substance put into your body to make clearer pictures during imaging tests.

creatinine
A waste product of muscles that is filtered out of blood into urine by the kidneys.

cytokines
Proteins made naturally in the body or in a lab that boost or activate the immune system.

cytokine therapy
Treatment with drugs that are cytokines—proteins made in a lab that boost or activate the immune system to fight cancer.

cytoreductive nephrectomy (CN)
Surgery to remove the primary tumor and the kidney when cancer that has spread to distant sites can't all be removed.

distant recurrence
Cancer that has come back after treatment and is found in a part of the body far from the first (primary) tumor.

deoxyribonucleic acid (DNA)
A chain of chemicals in cells that contains coded instructions for making and controlling cells.

first-line treatment
The first drug or set of drugs given to treat cancer.

gene
Coded instructions in cells for making new cells and controlling how cells behave.

Gerota's fascia
The outer layer of fibrous tissue that surrounds the kidney.

hereditary
Passed down from biological parent to child through genes.

histology
The structure of cells, tissue, and organs as viewed under a microscope.

imaging test
A test that makes pictures (images) of the insides of the body.

immune system
The body's natural defense against infection and disease.

immunotherapy
A treatment with drugs that helps the body find and destroy cancer cells.

kinase inhibitors
A type of targeted therapy.

laparoscopic surgery
Surgery that uses small tools and a laparoscope—a thin tube with a light and camera at the end—inserted through a few small cuts in the belly area.

local recurrence
Cancer that has come back after treatment in or near the same place as the first (primary) tumor.

lymph node
A small, bean-shaped, disease-fighting structure.

lymph node dissection
Surgery that removes some lymph nodes.

lymph vessels
Tubes that carry lymph—a clear fluid containing white blood cells that fight disease and infection—throughout the body and connect lymph nodes to one another.

magnetic resonance imaging (MRI)
A test that uses radio waves and powerful magnets to make pictures of the insides of the body.

mammalian target of rapamycin (mTOR)
A protein in cells that sends chemical signals for cell growth and survival.

metastasectomy
Surgery to remove tumors that formed far from the first site of cancer. Used to reduce cancer burden and to ease symptoms.

metastasis
The spread of cancer cells from the first tumor to another body part.

minimally invasive procedure
A procedure that uses small incisions or a tool placed into the opening of the body to reduce damage to body tissue.

monoclonal antibody (mAb)
A type of immune system protein made in a lab that can attach to substances in the body such as cancer cells. Can be a type of immunotherapy and a type of targeted therapy.

mTOR inhibitor
A drug that blocks the action of mTOR—a protein in cells that sends chemical signals for cell growth and survival. A type of targeted therapy.

mutation
An abnormal change.

nephrectomy
Surgery that removes a kidney.

non-clear cell RCC (nccRCC)
Subtypes of renal cell carcinoma (RCC) other than clear cell, based on how the cancer cells look when viewed with a microscope.

palliative care
Treatment for symptoms of a disease. Also sometimes called supportive care.

palliative nephrectomy
Surgery to remove the kidney to relieve symptoms caused by cancer.

palliative surgery
Surgery to relieve symptoms caused by the cancer.

papillary RCC (PRCC)
Most common type of RCC.

partial nephrectomy
Surgery to remove a tumor with part of the kidney.

pathologic stage (p)
A rating of the extent of cancer given after examining tissue removed during surgery.

primary treatment
The main treatment used to rid the body of cancer.

primary tumor
The first mass of cancer cells in the body.

prognosis
The likely course and outcome of a disease based on tests.

progression
The growth or spread of cancer after being tested or treated.

radiation therapy (RT)
A treatment that uses high-energy rays.

radical nephrectomy
Surgery that removes a tumor with the whole kidney, the fatty tissue around the kidney, and possibly the attached adrenal gland and nearby lymph nodes.

radiotracer
A substance that releases small amounts of energy (radiation) that is put into the body to make pictures clearer.

recurrence
The return of cancer after a cancer-free period.

relapse
The return of cancer after treatment. Also called a recurrence.

renal artery
The blood vessel that carries blood into the kidney.

renal cell carcinoma (RCC)
The most common type of kidney cancer. It starts in the cells that line the renal tubules—tiny tubes that filter blood and make urine.

renal pelvis
The space in the middle of the kidneys where urine collects before leaving the kidneys though long, thin tubes called ureters.

renal sarcoma
Cancer that starts in the blood vessels or connective tissue of the kidneys.

renal tubules
Tiny tubes in the kidneys that filter blood and make urine from the waste and extra water filtered out of blood.

renal vein
The blood vessel that carries clean blood out of the kidney.

resectable
Cancer that can be removed with surgery.

resection
Surgery to remove a tumor.

side effect
An unhealthy or unpleasant physical or emotional response to treatment

staging
The process of rating and describing the extent of cancer in the body.

stereotactic body radiation therapy (SBRT)
Radiation therapy given in higher doses to smaller areas over 1 to 5 sessions of treatment.

supportive care
Health care that includes symptom relief but not cancer treatment. Also called palliative care or best supportive care.

surveillance
Monitors for the return of cancer.

systemic therapy
Drug treatment that works throughout the body.

targeted therapy
A drug treatment that targets and attacks specific cancer cells

tumor
An abnormal mass of cells.

tyrosine kinase
A type of protein in cells that is important for many cell functions, such as sending signals for cell growth and survival.

tyrosine kinase inhibitor (TKI)
A targeted therapy that blocks the action of tyrosine kinases—proteins in cells that send signals for cells to grow, divide, and survive.

ultrasound (US)
A test that uses sound waves to take pictures of the insides of the body.

unresectable
Cancer that can't be removed by surgery.

ureter
A long, thin tube that carries urine from the kidney to the bladder.

urethra
The tube that carries urine from the bladder to outside the body.

urinalysis
A test that assesses the content of urine using a microscope and chemical tests.

urinary system
The group of organs that removes waste from the body in the form of urine. It is made up of the kidneys, ureters, bladder, and urethra.

urologist
A doctor who is an expert in treating diseases of the urinary system in both sexes and sex organs in those assigned male at birth.

vascular endothelial growth factor (VEGF)
A protein that binds to cells that form blood vessels.

vena cava
The main, large vein that carries blood back to the heart.

von Hippel-Lindau (VHL) disease
VHL gene helps control cell growth, cell division, and other important cell functions.

NCCN Contributors

This patient guide is based on the NCCN Clinical Practice Guidelines in Oncology (NCCN Guidelines®) for Kidney Cancer, Version 2.2025. It was adapted, reviewed, and published with help from the following people:

Dorothy A. Shead, MS
Senior Director
Patient Information Operations

Tanya Fischer, MEd, MSLIS
Senior Medical Writer

Susan Kidney
Senior Graphic Design Specialist

The NCCN Clinical Practice Guidelines in Oncology (NCCN Guidelines®) for Kidney Cancer, Version 2.2025 were developed by the following NCCN Panel Members:

*Robert J. Motzer, MD/Chair
Memorial Sloan Kettering Cancer Center

Eric Jonasch, MD/Vice-chair
The University of Texas
MD Anderson Cancer Center

Neeraj Agarwal, MD
Huntsman Cancer Institute
at the University of Utah

Ajjai Alva, MBBS
University of Michigan Rogel Cancer Center

Hilary Bagshaw, MD
Stanford Cancer Institute

*Michael Baine, MD, PhD
Fred & Pamela Buffet Cancer Center

Kathryn Beckermann, MD, PhD
Vanderbilt-Ingram Cancer Center

Maria I. Carlo, MD
Memorial Sloan Kettering Cancer Center

Toni K. Choueiri, MD
Dana-Farber/Brigham and Women's
Cancer Center | Mass General Cancer Center

Brian A. Costello, MD, MS
Mayo Clinic Comprehensive Cancer Center

Ithaar H. Derweesh, MD
UC San Diego Moores Cancer Center

Arpita Desai, MD
UCSF Helen Diller Family
Comprehensive Cancer Center

Yasser Ged, MBBS
Johns Hopkins Kimmel
Cancer

Saby George, MD
Roswell Park Comprehensive Cancer Center

Nikhil Gopal, MD
St. Jude Children's Research Hospital/
The University of Tennessee
Health Science Center

John L. Gore, MD, MS
Fred Hutchinson Cancer Center

Andrew Gunn, MD
O'Neal Comprehensive
Cancer Center at UAB

Naomi Haas, MD
Abramson Cancer Center
at the University of Pennsylvania

Michael Johnson, MD ω
Siteman Cancer Center at Barnes-
Jewish Hospital and Washington
University School of Medicine

Payal Kapur, MD
UT Southwestern Simmons
Comprehensive Cancer Center

Jennifer King, MD
Indiana University Melvin and Bren Simon
Comprehensive Cancer Center

Christos Kyriakopoulos, MD
University of Wisconsin
Carbone Cancer Center

*Elaine T. Lam, MD
University of Colorado Cancer Center

Primo N. Lara Jr., MD
UC Davis Comprehensive Cancer Center

Clayton Lau, MD
City of Hope National Medical Center

Bryan Lewis
KidneyCAN

David C. Madoff, MD
Yale Cancer Center/Smilow Cancer Hospital

*Brandon Manley, MD
Moffitt Cancer Center

M. Dror Michaelson, MD, PhD
Dana-Farber/Brigham and Women's
Cancer Center | Mass General Cancer Center

Amir Mortazavi, MD
The Ohio State University Comprehensive
Cancer Center - James Cancer Hospital
and Solove Research Institute

Lee Ponsky, MD
Case Comprehensive Cancer Center/
University Hospitals Seidman Cancer Center
and Cleveland Clinic Taussig Cancer Institute

Sundhar Ramalingam, MD
Duke Cancer Institute

Brian Shuch, MD
UCLA Jonsson Comprehensive
Cancer Center

Jeffrey Sosman, MD
Robert H. Lurie Comprehensive Cancer
Center of Northwestern University

Randy F. Sweis, MD
The UChicago Medicine
Comprehensive Cancer Center

Matthew Zibelman, MD
Fox Chase Cancer Center

NCCN

Ryan Schonfeld, BA
Guidelines Coordinator

MaryElizabeth Stein, PhD
Associate Scientist/Medical Writer

* Reviewed this patient guide. For disclosures, visit NCCN.org/disclosures.

NCCN Cancer Centers

Abramson Cancer Center
at the University of Pennsylvania
Philadelphia, Pennsylvania
800.789.7366 • pennmedicine.org/cancer

Case Comprehensive Cancer Center/
University Hospitals Seidman Cancer Center and
Cleveland Clinic Taussig Cancer Institute
Cleveland, Ohio
UH Seidman Cancer Center
800.641.2422 • uhhospitals.org/services/cancer-services
CC Taussig Cancer Institute
866.223.8100 • my.clevelandclinic.org/departments/cancer
Case CCC
216.844.8797 • case.edu/cancer

City of Hope National Medical Center
Duarte, California
800.826.4673 • cityofhope.org

Dana-Farber/Brigham and Women's Cancer Center |
Mass General Cancer Center
Boston, Massachusetts
877.442.3324 • youhaveus.org
617.726.5130 • massgeneral.org/cancer-center

Duke Cancer Institute
Durham, North Carolina
888.275.3853 • dukecancerinstitute.org

Fox Chase Cancer Center
Philadelphia, Pennsylvania
888.369.2427 • foxchase.org

Fred & Pamela Buffett Cancer Center
Omaha, Nebraska
402.559.5600 • unmc.edu/cancercenter

Fred Hutchinson Cancer Center
Seattle, Washington
206.667.5000 • fredhutch.org

Huntsman Cancer Institute at the University of Utah
Salt Lake City, Utah
800.824.2073 • healthcare.utah.edu/huntsmancancerinstitute

Indiana University Melvin and Bren Simon
Comprehensive Cancer Center
Indianapolis, Indiana
888.600.4822 • www.cancer.iu.edu

Johns Hopkins Kimmel Cancer Center
Baltimore, Maryland
410.955.8964
www.hopkinskimmelcancercenter.org

Mayo Clinic Comprehensive Cancer Center
Phoenix/Scottsdale, Arizona
Jacksonville, Florida
Rochester, Minnesota
480.301.8000 • Arizona
904.953.0853 • Florida
507.538.3270 • Minnesota
mayoclinic.org/cancercenter

Memorial Sloan Kettering Cancer Center
New York, New York
800.525.2225 • mskcc.org

Moffitt Cancer Center
Tampa, Florida
888.663.3488 • moffitt.org

O'Neal Comprehensive Cancer Center at UAB
Birmingham, Alabama
800.822.0933 • uab.edu/onealcancercenter

Robert H. Lurie Comprehensive Cancer Center
of Northwestern University
Chicago, Illinois
866.587.4322 • cancer.northwestern.edu

Roswell Park Comprehensive Cancer Center
Buffalo, New York
877.275.7724 • roswellpark.org

Siteman Cancer Center at Barnes-Jewish Hospital
and Washington University School of Medicine
St. Louis, Missouri
800.600.3606 • siteman.wustl.edu

St. Jude Children's Research Hospital/
The University of Tennessee Health Science Center
Memphis, Tennessee
866.278.5833 • stjude.org
901.448.5500 • uthsc.edu

Stanford Cancer Institute
Stanford, California
877.668.7535 • cancer.stanford.edu

The Ohio State University Comprehensive Cancer Center -
James Cancer Hospital and Solove Research Institute
Columbus, Ohio
800.293.5066 • cancer.osu.edu

The UChicago Medicine Comprehensive Cancer Center
Chicago, Illinois
773.702.1000 • uchicagomedicine.org/cancer

The University of Texas MD Anderson Cancer Center
Houston, Texas
844.269.5922 • mdanderson.org

UC Davis Comprehensive Cancer Center
Sacramento, California
916.734.5959 • 800.770.9261
health.ucdavis.edu/cancer

UC San Diego Moores Cancer Center
La Jolla, California
858.822.6100 • cancer.ucsd.edu

UCLA Jonsson Comprehensive Cancer Center
Los Angeles, California
310.825.5268 • uclahealth.org/cancer

UCSF Helen Diller Family
Comprehensive Cancer Center
San Francisco, California
800.689.8273 • cancer.ucsf.edu

University of Colorado Cancer Center
Aurora, Colorado
720.848.0300 • coloradocancercenter.org

University of Michigan Rogel Cancer Center
Ann Arbor, Michigan
800.865.1125 • rogelcancercenter.org

University of Wisconsin Carbone Cancer Center
Madison, Wisconsin
608.265.1700 • uwhealth.org/cancer

UT Southwestern Simmons
Comprehensive Cancer Center
Dallas, Texas
214.648.3111 • utsouthwestern.edu/simmons

Vanderbilt-Ingram Cancer Center
Nashville, Tennessee
877.936.8422 • vicc.org

Yale Cancer Center/Smilow Cancer Hospital
New Haven, Connecticut
855.4.SMILOW • yalecancercenter.org

share with us.

Take our survey and help make the NCCN Guidelines for Patients better for everyone!

NCCN.org/patients/comments

Index

Made in the USA
Monee, IL
25 June 2025

19603852R00050